CELIAC DISEASE DIET COOKBOOK FOR NEWLY DIAGNOSED

Delicious Gluten-free Recipes and Weekly Meals with Ideal Guidance to all Nutritional Requirements

TABLE OF CONTENTS

CHAPTER 1: INTRODUCTION

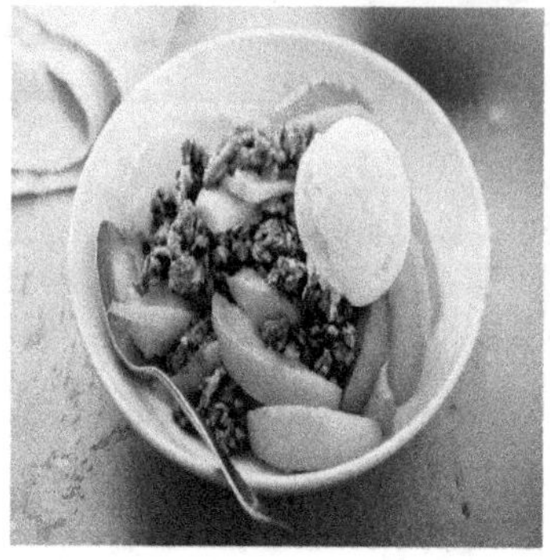

Imagine going on a one-of-a-kind voyage where the kitchen becomes your compass and your guide in a world flavored with gastronomic delights. Welcome to the "Celiac Cuisine Chronicles," a story written for people who have only recently discovered the complexities of living with Celiac Disease. Allow the aromatic whispers of gluten-free possibilities to enchant your senses and guide you through a newfound culinary experience as you flip through the pages of this cookbook. We'll turn dietary obstacles into a wonderful symphony of flavor, demonstrating that living a gluten-free lifestyle can be not only healthful but also a celebration of gourmet joy. Prepare to savor the enchantment of each recipe as we weave a wonderful story of health, flavor and a gluten-free life.

UNDERSTANDING CELIAC DISEASE

Celiac disease is a unique autoimmune condition that demands our attention as a subtle but significant disruptor of well-being. It is mostly caused by gluten sensitivity, a protein present in wheat, barley and rye. Consider the body to be a diligent gatekeeper, initiating an immune response against gluten by mistake causing harm to the small intestine.

This journey into the complexities of Celiac Disease entails not only decoding the biochemical details but also comprehending the tremendous impact on daily living. Each aspect reveals a new layer of obstacles and achievements, from identifying hidden gluten sources to navigating the social milieu of dining out.

Let us unravel the threads that connect symptoms, diagnosis, and the critical significance of a gluten-free diet as we delve into the scientific tapestry of Celiac Disease. We begin on a journey of understanding, encouraging people diagnosed as well as their advocates to traverse this gluten-free expedition with resilience, knowledge and a dash of culinary flare.

DIAGNOSIS AND ADJUSTING TO THE NEWS

Receiving a Celiac Disease diagnosis can be an unexpected diversion in life's journey, necessitating both mental and lifestyle changes. A combination of blood tests, genetic testing and a small intestine biopsy is frequently used in the diagnosis process. When the diagnosis is verified feelings may range from relief at finally understanding symptoms to the difficulty of adapting to a gluten-free lifestyle.

Adjusting to the news necessitates not only a change in food but also a shift in thinking. It's time to embrace your newfound health information and commit to a gluten-free lifestyle. Support networks, both within the medical community and among those living with Celiac Disease, become indispensable companions on this road of adaptation.

Remember that this shift isn't only about removing gluten; it's also about rediscovering the joy of food through a new lens. While it may appear difficult at first, adapting to life with Celiac Disease can lead to a healthier, more resilient and tasty chapter in your story with time and information.

TRANSITIONING TO A GLUTEN-FREE LIFESTYLE

Starting a gluten-free diet is a life-changing experience that goes beyond your plate. Consider this transition an opportunity to sample a diverse range of flavors and fuel your body with intention.

1. Educate Yourself: Learn about gluten-containing grains and their hidden sources. Read labels carefully and become acquainted with gluten-free alternatives.
2. Accept Whole Foods: Rediscover the ease and wholesomeness of naturally gluten-free foods such as fruits, vegetables, lean proteins and lentils. These will serve as the foundation for your new culinary artwork.
3. Explore Gluten-Free Grains: Delve into the world of gluten-free grains like quinoa, rice, millet and buckwheat. Experimenting with various grains allows you to expand your culinary horizons.
4. Join a Community: Seek help from local and online communities. Shared gluten-free journey experiences, insights and recipes can be invaluable companions.
5. Remodel Your Kitchen: Make your kitchen a gluten-free refuge by removing gluten-containing things. To avoid cross-contamination, purchase separate cooking utensils and cookware.
6. Communicate Clearly: When dining out or attending social functions, be clear about your dietary demands. This promotes comprehension and ensures a safe gluten-free experience.

CHAPTER 2: BREAKFASTS

Quinoa Breakfast Bowl:

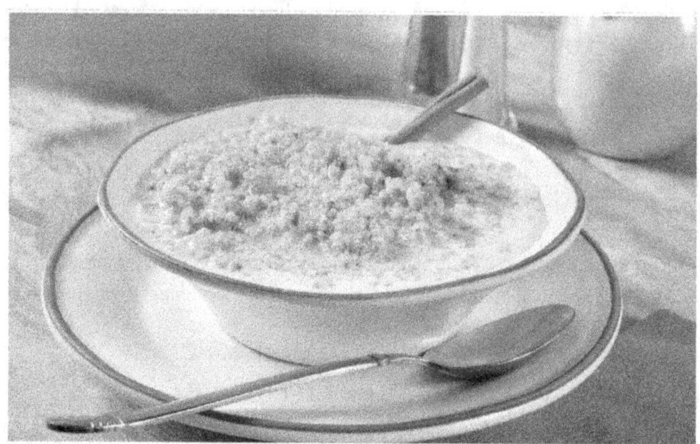

Ingredients:

- 1 cup quinoa
- 2 cups water
- 1 cup almond milk (or any milk of your choice)
- 1 tablespoon honey or maple syrup
- 1 teaspoon vanilla extract
- 1/2 teaspoon cinnamon
- Fresh fruits (e.g berries, banana slices)
- Nuts and seeds (e.g almonds, chia seeds)
- Greek yogurt or non-dairy alternative

Instructions:

1. Rinse quinoa under cold water.
2. In a medium saucepan, combine quinoa and water. Bring to a boil, then reduce heat, cover and simmer for 15 minutes or until quinoa is cooked and water is absorbed.

3. In a separate small saucepan, warm almond milk over low heat. Add honey or maple syrup, vanilla extract and cinnamon. Stir until well combined.

4. Once quinoa is cooked, fluff it with a fork and transfer to a bowl.

5. Pour the sweetened almond milk mixture over the quinoa and stir.

6. Top the quinoa with fresh fruits, nuts, seeds and a dollop of Greek yogurt or non-dairy alternative.

7. Enjoy your nutritious and delicious quinoa breakfast bowl!

Prep Time: Approximately 20 minutes

Gluten-Free Oatmeal with Fruit:

Ingredients:

- 1 cup gluten-free rolled oats
- 2 cups water
- 1 cup milk (dairy or non-dairy)
- 1 tablespoon honey or maple syrup
- 1/2 teaspoon vanilla extract
- Pinch of salt
- Fresh fruits (e.g berries, sliced banana)
- Nuts and seeds (e.g sliced almonds, chia seeds)
- Cinnamon for garnish

Instructions:

1. In a saucepan, combine gluten-free rolled oats and water. Bring to a boil, then reduce heat to medium-low and simmer for about 5-7 minutes or until oats are cooked to your liking.

2. Add milk to the oats and continue to cook, stirring frequently until the mixture reaches your desired consistency.

3. Stir in honey or maple syrup, vanilla extract and a pinch of salt. Mix well.

4. Remove the oatmeal from heat and transfer it to a bowl.

5. Top the oatmeal with fresh fruits, nuts and seeds.

6. Sprinkle it with cinnamon for added flavor.

7. Allow it to cool for a minute before serving.

8. Customize with additional toppings as desired.

Egg and Vegetable Scramble:

Ingredients:

- 1 frozen banana, sliced
- 1 cup frozen mixed berries (strawberries, blueberries, raspberries)
- 1/2 cup plain Greek yogurt or non-dairy alternative
- 1/2 cup almond milk or any milk of your choice
- 1 tablespoon chia seeds
- Toppings: Sliced fruits, granola, nuts, seeds, shredded coconut

Instructions:

1. In a blender, combine the frozen banana slices, frozen mixed berries, Greek yogurt, almond milk and chia seeds.

2. Blend until smooth and creamy. You may need to stop and scrape down the sides of the blender as needed.

3. Pour the smoothie into a bowl.

4. Arrange your desired toppings on top of the smoothie. Get creative with the presentation!

5. Serve immediately and enjoy your refreshing and nutritious smoothie bowl.

Smoothie Bowl:

Ingredients:

- 1 frozen banana, sliced
- 1 cup frozen mixed berries (strawberries, blueberries, raspberries)
- 1/2 cup plain Greek yogurt or non-dairy alternative
- 1/2 cup almond milk or any milk of your choice
- 1 tablespoon chia seeds

- Toppings: Sliced fruits, granola, nuts, seeds, shredded coconut

Instructions:

1. In a blender, combine the frozen banana slices, frozen mixed berries, Greek yogurt, almond milk and chia seeds.
2. Blend until smooth and creamy. You may need to stop and scrape down the sides of the blender as needed.
3. Pour the smoothie into a bowl.
4. Arrange your desired toppings on top of the smoothie. Get creative with the presentation!
5. Serve immediately and enjoy your refreshing and nutritious smoothie bowl.

Chia Seed Pudding:

Ingredients:

- 1/4 cup chia seeds
- 1 cup almond milk (or any milk of your choice)
- 1 tablespoon honey or maple syrup
- 1/2 teaspoon vanilla extract
- Fresh fruits for topping (e.g berries, sliced kiwi)
- Nuts and seeds for garnish (e.g sliced almonds, sunflower seeds)

Instructions:

1. In a bowl, mix chia seeds, almond milk, honey or maple syrup, and vanilla extract. Stir well to combine.
2. Cover the bowl and refrigerate the mixture for at least 2 hours or preferably overnight. This allows the chia seeds to absorb the liquid and create a pudding-like consistency.
3. After refrigeration, stir the chia pudding well to break up any clumps.
4. Spoon the chia pudding into serving bowls or glasses.
5. Top with fresh fruits and your choice of nuts or seeds for added texture and flavor.
6. Drizzle with a bit more honey or maple syrup if desired.

7. Serve chilled and enjoy your nutritious and satisfying chia seed pudding!

Gluten-Free Pancakes:

Ingredients:

- 1 cup gluten-free all-purpose flour
- 1 tablespoon sugar
- 1 teaspoon baking powder
- 1/2 teaspoon baking soda
- 1/4 teaspoon salt
- 1 cup buttermilk (or non-dairy alternative with 1 tablespoon of vinegar or lemon juice)
- 1 large egg
- 2 tablespoons melted butter (or oil for dairy-free option)
- 1 teaspoon vanilla extract

Instructions:

1. In a mixing bowl, whisk together gluten-free flour, sugar, baking powder, baking soda and salt.
2. In a separate bowl, whisk buttermilk, egg, melted butter and vanilla extract.
3. Pour the wet ingredients into the dry ingredients and stir until just combined. Do not overmix; a few lumps are okay.
4. Let the batter rest for 5-10 minutes to allow the gluten-free flour to absorb the liquid.
5. Heat a griddle or non-stick skillet over medium heat. Lightly grease with cooking spray or butter.
6. Pour 1/4 cup of batter onto the hot griddle for each pancake.
7. Cook until bubbles form on the surface, then flip and cook the other side until golden brown.
8. Repeat with the remaining batter.

9. Serve the gluten-free pancakes warm with your favorite toppings, such as maple syrup, fresh fruit or whipped cream.

Sweet Potato Hash:

Ingredients:
- 2 medium-sized sweet potatoes, peeled and diced into small cubes
- 1 red bell pepper, diced
- 1 yellow onion, finely chopped
- 2 cloves garlic, minced
- 2 tablespoons olive oil
- 1 teaspoon paprika
- 1/2 teaspoon cumin
- Salt and pepper to taste
- Fresh parsley or cilantro for garnish (optional)
- Fried or poached eggs for serving (optional)

Instructions:
1. Heat olive oil in a large skillet over medium heat.
2. Add the diced sweet potatoes to the skillet and cook for 5-7 minutes, stirring occasionally until they start to soften.
3. Add the diced red bell pepper and chopped onion to the skillet. Continue cooking for another 5-7 minutes until the vegetables are tender.
4. Stir in minced garlic, paprika, cumin, salt, and pepper. Cook for an additional 2 minutes to allow the flavors to meld.
5. Continue cooking and stirring occasionally until the sweet potatoes are golden brown and fully cooked.
6. Taste and adjust seasoning as needed.
7. Optional: Top with fresh parsley or cilantro for added freshness.
8. Serve the sweet potato hash as a side dish or as a base for fried or poached eggs.

Yogurt Parfait:

Ingredients:
- 1 cup Greek yogurt (or any yogurt of your choice)
- 2 tablespoons honey or maple syrup
- 1/2 cup granola
- 1/2 cup mixed berries (e.g strawberries, blueberries, raspberries)
- 1 tablespoon chia seeds (optional)

- Nuts or seeds for crunch (e.g sliced almonds, pumpkin seeds)

Instructions:

1. In a bowl, mix Greek yogurt with honey or maple syrup until well combined.
2. In serving glasses or bowls, layer the yogurt mixture, granola and mixed berries.
3. Repeat the layers until you reach the top, finishing with a dollop of yogurt on the top.
4. Sprinkle chia seeds over the parfait for added texture and nutritional benefits.
5. Top with nuts or seeds for an extra crunch.
6. Optionally, drizzle a little extra honey or maple syrup on top for sweetness.
7. Refrigerate for at least 30 minutes to allow the flavors to meld and the parfait to chill.
8. Before serving, give it a gentle stir to combine the layers.

Avocado Toast on Gluten-Free Bread:

Ingredients:

- 2 slices gluten-free bread
- 1 ripe avocado
- 1 tablespoon lemon juice
- Salt and pepper to taste
- Red pepper flakes for optional spice
- Optional toppings: Cherry tomatoes, radish slices, poached egg or feta cheese

Instructions:

1. Toast the gluten-free bread slices to your desired level of crispiness.
2. While the bread is toasting, cut the avocado in half, remove the pit and scoop the flesh into a bowl.
3. Mash the avocado with a fork and mix in lemon juice, salt and pepper. Adjust seasoning to taste.
4. Spread the mashed avocado evenly over the toasted gluten-free bread slices.
5. Optionally, top with red pepper flakes for a hint of spice.
6. Add additional toppings of your choice such as cherry tomatoes, radish slices, a poached egg or crumbled feta cheese.
7. Serve immediately and enjoy your tasty and nutritious avocado toast!

Baked Egg Cups:

Ingredients:

- 6 large eggs

- 1 cup spinach, chopped
- 1/2 cup cherry tomatoes, diced
- 1/4 cup feta cheese, crumbled
- Salt and pepper to taste
- Cooking spray or butter for greasing

Instructions:

1. Preheat your oven to 375°F (190°C). Grease a muffin tin with cooking spray or butter.
2. In a bowl, whisk the eggs until well beaten. Season with salt and pepper.
3. Divide the chopped spinach, diced cherry tomatoes, and crumbled feta cheese evenly among the muffin tin cups.
4. Pour the whisked eggs over the vegetables and cheese in each cup, filling them about 3/4 full.
5. Gently stir the mixture in each cup with a fork to ensure even distribution of ingredients.
6. Bake in the preheated oven for 15-20 minutes or until the eggs are set and slightly golden on top.
7. Remove the baked egg cups from the oven and let them cool for a few minutes.
8. Carefully run a knife around the edges of each cup and use a fork to lift them out.
9. Serve warm and enjoy your flavorful and protein-packed baked egg cups!

Rice Cake with Nut Butter and Banana:

Ingredients:

- 1 rice cake (choose a variety that fits your dietary preferences)
- 1-2 tablespoons of nut butter (peanut butter, almond butter etc.)
- 1 ripe banana, sliced
- Optional: Drizzle of honey or sprinkle of cinnamon

Instructions:

1. Place a rice cake on a plate or flat surface.
2. Spread a generous layer of nut butter over the rice cake. Ensure an even coating.
3. Arrange banana slices on top of the nut butter-covered rice cake.
4. Optional: Drizzle honey over the banana slices or sprinkle a bit of cinnamon for added flavor.
5. Serve immediately and enjoy your quick and satisfying rice cake with nut butter and banana!

CHAPTER 3: LUNCH AND DINNERS

Quinoa Salad with Grilled Chicken:

Ingredients:

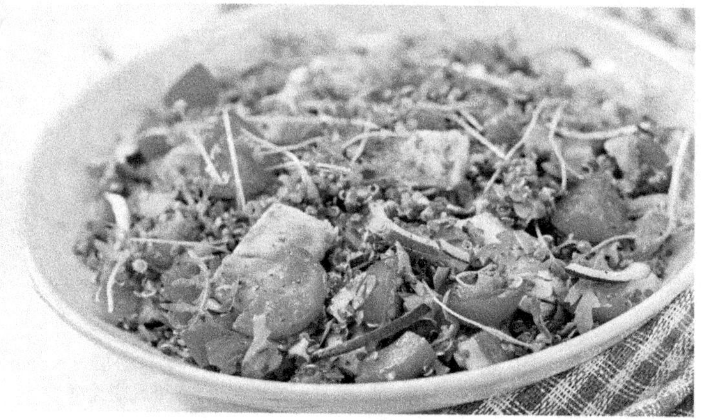

For the Salad:

- 1 cup quinoa, rinsed
- 2 cups water or chicken broth for cooking quinoa
- 1 pound boneless, skinless chicken breasts
- 1 tablespoon olive oil
- Salt and pepper to taste
- 1 cup cherry tomatoes, halved
- 1 cucumber, diced
- 1 bell pepper, diced
- 1/4 cup red onion, finely chopped
- 1/2 cup feta cheese, crumbled
- Fresh parsley, chopped for garnish

For the Dressing:

- 3 tablespoons olive oil
- 2 tablespoons balsamic vinegar
- 1 teaspoon Dijon mustard
- 1 clove garlic, minced
- Salt and pepper to taste

Instructions:

1. Prepare Quinoa:
   - In a saucepan, combine quinoa and water or chicken broth. Bring to a boil, then reduce heat, cover and simmer for 15 minutes or until quinoa is cooked. Fluff with a fork and let it cool.

2. Grill Chicken:
   - Preheat the grill or grill pan over medium-high heat.
   - Rub chicken breasts with olive oil and season with salt and pepper.
   - Grill the chicken for 6-8 minutes per side or until fully cooked. Let it rest for a few minutes before slicing.

3. Make the Dressing:
   - In a small bowl, whisk together olive oil, balsamic vinegar, Dijon mustard, minced garlic, salt and pepper. Set aside.

4. Assemble the Salad:
   - In a large bowl, combine cooked quinoa, cherry tomatoes, cucumber, bell pepper and red onion.
   - Add the grilled chicken slices on top.
   - Pour the dressing over the salad and toss everything together until well coated.
   - Sprinkle crumbled feta cheese and chopped fresh parsley on top.

5. Serve:
   - Serve the quinoa salad with grilled chicken immediately or refrigerate for later.

Gluten-Free Wrap with Turkey and Avocado:

Ingredients:

- 1 gluten-free tortilla/wrap
- 4 ounces sliced turkey breast
- 1/2 avocado, sliced
- 1/4 cup cucumber, thinly sliced
- 1/4 cup shredded lettuce
- 1 tablespoon mayonnaise or Greek yogurt
- 1 teaspoon Dijon mustard
- Salt and pepper to taste

Instructions:

1. Prepare the Wrap:
   - Lay the gluten-free tortilla on a flat surface.
2. Layer the Ingredients:
   - Spread mayonnaise or Greek yogurt over the center of the tortilla.
   - Arrange sliced turkey evenly over the sauce.
   - Place avocado slices, cucumber and shredded lettuce on top of the turkey.
3. Season and Dress:
   - Drizzle Dijon mustard over the fillings.
   - Sprinkle salt and pepper to taste.
4. Wrap It Up:
   - Fold the sides of the tortilla towards the center.
   - Starting from the bottom, tightly roll the tortilla to create a wrap.
5. Slice and Serve:
   - Slice the wrap diagonally into halves or enjoy it whole.
6. Optional: Warm It Up:
   - If desired, you can warm the gluten-free wrap in a skillet for a few minutes on each side.

Mango Salsa Chicken Lettuce Wraps:

Ingredients:

For the Chicken:
- 1 pound boneless, skinless chicken breasts
- 1 tablespoon olive oil
- 1 teaspoon ground cumin
- 1 teaspoon chili powder
- Salt and pepper to taste

For the Mango Salsa:
- 1 ripe mango, peeled, pitted, and diced
- 1/2 red onion, finely chopped
- 1 jalapeño, seeds removed and finely chopped
- 1/4 cup fresh cilantro, chopped
- Juice of 1 lime
- Salt to taste

For Assembling:
- Large lettuce leaves (butter lettuce or iceberg)
- Avocado slices (optional)

Instructions:
1. **Cook the Chicken:**
   - In a skillet, heat olive oil over medium-high heat.
   - Season chicken breasts with cumin, chili powder, salt and pepper.
   - Cook the chicken for about 6-8 minutes per side or until fully cooked. Let it rest for a few minutes, then shred.
2. Prepare the Mango Salsa:
   - In a bowl, combine diced mango, chopped red onion, jalapeno, cilantro, lime juice and salt. Mix well.
3. Assemble the Lettuce Wraps:
   - Take a large lettuce leaf, spoon some shredded chicken onto it.
   - Top with mango salsa and avocado slices if desired.
4. Serve:
   - Arrange the assembled mango salsa chicken lettuce wraps on a plate.

Greek Chickpea Salad:

Ingredients:
- 1 can (15 oz) chickpeas, drained and rinsed

- 1 cucumber, diced
- 1 cup cherry tomatoes, halved
- 1/2 red onion, finely chopped
- 1/2 cup Kalamata olives, sliced
- 1/2 cup feta cheese, crumbled
- 1/4 cup fresh parsley, chopped

For the Dressing:

- 3 tablespoons extra virgin olive oil
- 1 tablespoon red wine vinegar
- 1 teaspoon dried oregano
- Salt and pepper to taste
- Optional: Lemon juice for extra freshness

Instructions:

1. Prepare Chickpeas:
   - Drain and rinse the canned chickpeas thoroughly.
2. Assemble Salad:
   - In a large bowl, combine chickpeas, diced cucumber, cherry tomatoes, chopped red onion, sliced Kalamata olives, feta cheese and fresh parsley.
3. Make the Dressing:
   - In a small bowl, whisk together olive oil, red wine vinegar, dried oregano, salt and pepper. Adjust seasoning to taste.
   - Optionally, squeeze fresh lemon juice into the dressing for added brightness.
4. Dress the Salad:
   - Pour the dressing over the salad ingredients.
5. Toss Gently:
   - Gently toss the salad until all ingredients are well coated with the dressing.
6. Chill:

- o Refrigerate the Greek Chickpea Salad for at least 30 minutes before serving to allow the flavors to meld.

Sweet Potato and Black Bean Bowl:

Ingredients:

- 2 medium-sized sweet potatoes, peeled and diced
- 1 can (15 oz) black beans, drained and rinsed
- 1 cup corn kernels (fresh, frozen or canned)
- 1 red bell pepper, diced
- 1 tablespoon olive oil
- 1 teaspoon ground cumin
- 1 teaspoon chili powder
- Salt and pepper to taste

For the Lime-Cilantro Dressing:

- Juice of 2 limes
- 3 tablespoons olive oil
- 2 tablespoons fresh cilantro, chopped
- 1 clove garlic, minced
- Salt and pepper to taste

Optional Toppings:

- Avocado slices
- Greek yogurt or sour cream
- Salsa

Instructions:

1. Roast Sweet Potatoes:
   - o Preheat the oven to 400°F (200°C).
   - o Toss diced sweet potatoes with olive oil, ground cumin, chili powder, salt and pepper.

    ○ Spread on a baking sheet and roast for 20-25 minutes or until sweet potatoes are tender and slightly crispy.

2. Prepare Black Beans and Vegetables:
    ○ In a skillet over medium heat, combine black beans, corn and diced red bell pepper. Cook until heated through.

3. Make the Lime-Cilantro Dressing:
    ○ In a small bowl, whisk together lime juice, olive oil, chopped cilantro, minced garlic, salt and pepper.

4. Assemble the Bowl:
    ○ In serving bowls, layer the roasted sweet potatoes, black bean and vegetable mixture.
    ○ Drizzle the lime-cilantro dressing over the top.

5. Optional Toppings:
    ○ Add optional toppings like avocado slices, a dollop of Greek yogurt or sour cream and salsa.

Gluten-Free Quiche with Spinach and Feta:

Ingredients:

For the Gluten-Free Crust:

- 1 1/2 cups gluten-free all-purpose flour
- 1/2 cup cold unsalted butter, cubed
- 1/4 cup ice-cold water
- 1/2 teaspoon salt

For the Filling:

- 1 cup fresh spinach, chopped
- 1/2 cup feta cheese, crumbled
- 1/4 cup grated Parmesan cheese
- 4 large eggs
- 1 cup milk (dairy or non-dairy)

- Salt and pepper to taste
- Pinch of nutmeg (optional)

Instructions:

1. Prepare the Gluten-Free Crust:
   - In a food processor, pulse the gluten-free flour and cold butter until it resembles coarse crumbs.
   - Add cold water and salt, pulsing until the dough comes together.
   - Press the dough into the bottom of a pie dish to form the crust. Place it in the refrigerator while preparing the filling.
2. Preheat Oven:
   - Preheat your oven to 375°F (190°C).
3. Prepare the Filling:
   - In a skillet, sauté chopped spinach until wilted. Remove excess moisture by pressing the spinach between paper towels.
   - In a bowl, whisk together eggs, milk, salt, pepper and nutmeg (if using).
4. Assemble the Quiche:
   - Sprinkle crumbled feta cheese and grated Parmesan over the chilled crust.
   - Spread the sautéed spinach evenly over the cheese.
   - Pour the egg mixture over the spinach and cheese.
5. Bake:
   - Bake in the preheated oven for 35-40 minutes or until the quiche is set and golden brown.
6. Cool and Serve:
   - Allow the quiche to cool for a few minutes before slicing.

Caprese Skewers:

Ingredients:

- Cherry tomatoes
- Fresh mozzarella balls (bocconcini)

- Fresh basil leaves
- Balsamic glaze (store-bought or homemade)
- Extra virgin olive oil
- Salt and pepper to taste
- Wooden skewers

Instructions:

1. Prepare Ingredients:
   - Rinse cherry tomatoes and fresh basil leaves.
   - If needed, drain the mozzarella balls.
2. Assemble Skewers:
   - Thread one cherry tomato, one fresh mozzarella ball and one basil leaf onto each wooden skewer.
3. Arrange on Platter:
   - Arrange the assembled skewers on a serving platter.
4. Season:
   - Drizzle extra virgin olive oil over the skewers.
   - Sprinkle it with salt and pepper to taste.
5. Drizzle with Balsamic Glaze:
   - Drizzle balsamic glaze over the skewers. If you don't have balsamic glaze, you can reduce balsamic vinegar on the stovetop until it thickens.

Salmon Salad with Citrus Dressing:

Ingredients:

For the Salmon:

- 4 salmon filets
- 1 tablespoon olive oil
- Salt and pepper to taste
- 1 teaspoon paprika
- 1 teaspoon dried dill (or 1 tablespoon fresh dill)

For the Salad:

- Mixed salad greens (e.g arugula, spinach, watercress)
- 1 cucumber, sliced
- 1 cup cherry tomatoes, halved
- 1/4 red onion, thinly sliced
- Avocado slices (optional)

For the Citrus Dressing:

- Juice of 2 oranges
- Juice of 1 lemon
- 3 tablespoons extra virgin olive oil
- 1 tablespoon honey or maple syrup
- Salt and pepper to taste

Instructions:

1. **Preheat Oven:**
   - Preheat the oven to 400°F (200°C).
2. Prepare Salmon:
   - Place salmon filets on a baking sheet.
   - Drizzle with olive oil and season with salt, pepper, paprika and dried dill.
   - Bake for 12-15 minutes or until the salmon is cooked through and flakes easily with a fork.
3. Make Citrus Dressing:
   - In a bowl, whisk together orange juice, lemon juice, extra virgin olive oil, honey or maple syrup, salt and pepper. Set aside.
4. Assemble Salad:
   - In a large bowl, toss together mixed salad greens, sliced cucumber, halved cherry tomatoes and thinly sliced red onion.
   - Optional: Add avocado slices to the salad.
5. Flake Salmon:

- Once the salmon is cooked, use a fork to gently flake it into bite-sized pieces.

6. Combine Salad and Salmon:
   - Add the flaked salmon to the salad mixture.
7. Drizzle with Dressing:
   - Drizzle the citrus dressing over the salad and salmon. Toss gently to combine.
8. Serve:
   - Serve the salmon salad with citrus dressing immediately.

Vegetarian Rice Paper Rolls:

Ingredients:

For the Rice Paper Rolls:

- 8-10 rice paper wrappers
- 1 cup rice vermicelli noodles, cooked and cooled
- 1 cucumber, julienned
- 1 carrot, julienned
- 1 red bell pepper, thinly sliced
- 1 avocado, sliced
- Fresh herbs (mint, cilantro, basil)
- Lettuce leaves

For the Dipping Sauce:

- 1/4 cup soy sauce or tamari (for gluten-free)
- 2 tablespoons hoisin sauce
- 1 tablespoon rice vinegar
- 1 teaspoon sesame oil
- 1 teaspoon honey or maple syrup
- 1 clove garlic, minced
- Crushed peanuts for garnish (optional)

Instructions:

1. Prepare Ingredients:
   - Cook rice vermicelli noodles according to package instructions and let them cool.
   - Julienne cucumber, carrot and thinly slice the red bell pepper.
   - Slice avocado and prepare fresh herbs and lettuce leaves.
2. Soak Rice Paper Wrappers:
   - Fill a shallow dish with warm water.
   - Dip one rice paper wrapper into the water for about 10-15 seconds until it becomes soft and pliable.
3. Assemble the Rice Paper Rolls:
   - Place the softened rice paper on a clean surface.
   - In the center, add a small amount of rice vermicelli noodles, cucumber, carrot, red bell pepper, avocado slices, fresh herbs and a lettuce leaf.
4. Roll the Rice Paper:
   - Fold the sides of the rice paper over the filling, then roll it tightly from the bottom to the top, sealing the edge.
5. Repeat:
   - Repeat the process with the remaining rice paper wrappers and filling ingredients.
6. Prepare Dipping Sauce:
   - In a small bowl, whisk together soy sauce or tamari, hoisin sauce, rice vinegar, sesame oil, honey or maple syrup and minced garlic.
7. Serve:
   - Serve the vegetarian rice paper rolls with the dipping sauce.

Stuffed Bell Peppers:

Ingredients:

- 4 large bell peppers (any color)

- 1 cup cooked quinoa or rice
- 1 pound ground meat (beef, turkey or plant-based alternative)
- 1 onion, finely chopped
- 2 cloves garlic, minced
- 1 can (15 oz) black beans, drained and rinsed
- 1 cup corn kernels (fresh, frozen or canned)
- 1 cup diced tomatoes
- 1 teaspoon ground cumin
- 1 teaspoon chili powder
- Salt and pepper to taste
- 1 cup shredded cheese (cheddar, Monterey Jack or your choice)
- Fresh cilantro or parsley for garnish (optional)

Instructions:

1. Preheat Oven:
   - Preheat the oven to 375°F (190°C).
2. Prepare Bell Peppers:
   - Cut the tops off the bell peppers and remove seeds and membranes.
   - If needed, slice a small portion from the bottom of each pepper to make them stand upright.
3. Cook the Meat:
   - In a skillet over medium heat, cook the ground meat until browned. Drain excess fat if needed.
4. Sauté Vegetables:
   - In the same skillet, sauté chopped onion and minced garlic until softened.
   - Add diced tomatoes, black beans, corn, ground cumin, chili powder, salt and pepper. Cook for an additional 5 minutes.
5. Combine:
   - In a large bowl, combine the cooked quinoa or rice with the sautéed meat and vegetable mixture. Mix well.

6. Stuff Bell Peppers:

    o Stuff each bell pepper with the quinoa or rice mixture, pressing down gently.

    o Top each stuffed pepper with shredded cheese.

7. Bake:

    o Place the stuffed bell peppers in a baking dish.

    o Bake in the preheated oven for 25-30 minutes or until the peppers are tender.

8. Garnish and Serve:

    o Garnish with fresh cilantro or parsley if desired.

    o Serve the stuffed bell peppers hot.

Gluten-Free Margherita Pizza:

Ingredients:

For the Gluten-Free Pizza Crust:

- 2 1/2 cups gluten-free all-purpose flour
- 1 teaspoon xanthan gum (if your flour blend doesn't contain it)
- 1 packet (2 1/4 teaspoons) active dry yeast
- 1 teaspoon sugar
- 1 cup warm water (110°F/43°C)
- 2 tablespoons olive oil
- 1 teaspoon salt

For the Pizza Toppings:

- 1/2 cup pizza sauce
- 1-2 large tomatoes, thinly sliced
- Fresh mozzarella cheese, sliced
- Fresh basil leaves
- Extra virgin olive oil
- Salt and pepper to taste

Instructions:

1. Prepare the Pizza Dough:
   - In a small bowl, combine warm water, sugar, and active dry yeast. Let it sit for about 5 minutes until frothy.
   - In a large mixing bowl, combine gluten-free flour, xanthan gum (if needed), olive oil, and salt. Add the yeast mixture and mix until a dough forms.
   - Knead the dough for a few minutes until smooth. If it's too sticky, add a bit more flour.
   - Cover the bowl with a clean kitchen towel and let the dough rise for about 1 hour or until it doubles in size.
2. Preheat Oven:
   - Preheat your oven to 425°F (220°C).
3. Roll Out the Dough:
   - Place the dough on a piece of parchment paper. Dust the top with gluten-free flour and roll it out to your desired thickness.
4. Assemble the Pizza:
   - Transfer the parchment paper with the rolled-out dough onto a baking sheet or pizza stone.
   - Spread pizza sauce evenly over the crust.
   - Arrange tomato slices and fresh mozzarella on top.
   - Season with salt and pepper.
   - Drizzle with a bit of extra virgin olive oil.
5. Bake:
   - Bake in the preheated oven for 15-20 minutes or until the crust is golden and the cheese is melted and bubbly.
6. Finish with Fresh Basil:
   - Remove from the oven and sprinkle fresh basil leaves over the hot pizza.
7. Slice and Serve:
   - Slice the gluten-free Margherita pizza and serve immediately.

Lemon Garlic Herb Chicken:

Ingredients:

- 4 boneless, skinless chicken breasts
- 4 tablespoons olive oil
- 4 cloves garlic, minced
- Zest of 1 lemon
- Juice of 1 lemon
- 1 teaspoon dried thyme
- 1 teaspoon dried rosemary
- Salt and pepper to taste
- Fresh parsley for garnish

Instructions:

1. Preheat Oven:
   - Preheat your oven to 400°F (200°C).
2. Prepare Chicken:
   - Pat the chicken breasts dry with paper towels.
   - Season both sides with salt and pepper.
3. Make the Marinade:
   - In a bowl, whisk together olive oil, minced garlic, lemon zest, lemon juice, dried thyme and dried rosemary.
4. Marinate Chicken:
   - Place the chicken breasts in a zip-top bag or a shallow dish.
   - Pour the marinade over the chicken, making sure each piece is well coated.
   - Allow the chicken to marinate for at least 30 minutes to enhance the flavors.
5. Cook Chicken:
   - Heat an oven-safe skillet over medium-high heat.

- o Add a bit of olive oil to the skillet.
    - o Sear the chicken breasts for 2-3 minutes on each side until golden brown.
6. Finish in the Oven:
    - o Transfer the skillet to the preheated oven.
    - o Bake for 20-25 minutes or until the chicken is cooked through (internal temperature reaches 165°F or 74°C).
7. Garnish and Serve:
    - o Remove from the oven and let the chicken rest for a few minutes.
    - o Garnish with fresh parsley before serving.

Gluten-Free Spaghetti Bolognese:

Ingredients:

- **1 pound gluten-free** spaghetti
- 1 tablespoon olive oil
- 1 onion, finely chopped
- 2 carrots, diced
- 2 celery stalks, diced
- 3 cloves garlic, minced
- 1 pound ground beef or ground turkey
- 1 can (28 oz) crushed tomatoes
- 1/2 cup red wine (optional)
- 1 teaspoon dried oregano
- 1 teaspoon dried basil
- Salt and pepper to taste
- 1/4 teaspoon red pepper flakes (optional, for heat)
- Fresh basil or parsley for garnish
- Grated Parmesan or nutritional yeast for topping (optional)

Instructions:

1. Cook Gluten-Free Spaghetti:

- ○ Cook the gluten-free spaghetti according to the package instructions. Drain and set aside.

2. Prepare Bolognese Sauce:
   - ○ In a large skillet or pot, heat olive oil over medium heat.
   - ○ Add chopped onion, diced carrots and diced celery. Sauté until softened.

3. Cook Ground Meat:
   - ○ Add minced garlic and ground meat (beef or turkey) to the skillet. Cook until the meat is browned.

4. Add Crushed Tomatoes and Seasoning:
   - ○ Pour in the crushed tomatoes and red wine (if using). Stir to combine.
   - ○ Season with dried oregano, dried basil, salt, pepper and red pepper flakes if you want a bit of heat.

5. Simmer:
   - ○ Bring the sauce to a simmer, then reduce the heat to low. Let it simmer for at least 20-30 minutes to allow the flavors to meld.

6. Adjust Seasoning:
   - ○ Taste and adjust seasoning as needed. If the sauce is too thick, you can add a bit of water or beef/turkey broth.

7. Serve:
   - ○ Spoon the Bolognese sauce over the cooked gluten-free spaghetti.

Teriyaki Salmon with Stir-Fried Vegetables:

Ingredients:

For Teriyaki Salmon:

- 4 salmon filets
- 1/2 cup teriyaki sauce
- 2 tablespoons soy sauce
- 2 tablespoons honey
- 1 tablespoon rice vinegar

- 2 teaspoons sesame oil
- 2 cloves garlic, minced
- 1 teaspoon grated ginger
- Sesame seeds and chopped green onions for garnish

For Stir-Fried Vegetables:

- 2 tablespoons vegetable oil
- 1 broccoli crown, cut into florets
- 1 bell pepper, thinly sliced
- 1 carrot, julienned
- 1 zucchini, sliced
- 3 green onions, sliced
- 2 cloves garlic, minced
- 1 tablespoon soy sauce
- 1 teaspoon sesame oil
- Sesame seeds for garnish

Instructions:

For Teriyaki Salmon:

1. Prepare Marinade:
   - In a bowl, whisk together teriyaki sauce, soy sauce, honey, rice vinegar, sesame oil, minced garlic and grated ginger.
2. Marinate Salmon:
   - Place salmon filets in a shallow dish or a zip-top bag. Pour half of the teriyaki marinade over the salmon. Reserve the other half for later.
   - Marinate the salmon in the refrigerator for at least 30 minutes.
3. Cook Salmon:
   - Preheat the oven to 400°F (200°C).
   - Place the marinated salmon filets on a baking sheet lined with parchment paper.

- Bake for 15-20 minutes or until the salmon is cooked through, basting with the reserved teriyaki marinade halfway through.
  - Optionally, broil for the last 2-3 minutes for a caramelized finish.
  - Garnish the salmon with sesame seeds and chopped green onions.

For Stir-Fried Vegetables:

1. Sauté Vegetables:
   - In a wok or large skillet, heat vegetable oil over medium-high heat.
   - Add sliced bell pepper, julienned carrot, sliced zucchini and broccoli florets. Stir-fry for 3-5 minutes or until the vegetables are crisp-tender.
2. Add Aromatics:
   - Add minced garlic and sliced green onions to the vegetables. Stir-fry for an additional 1-2 minutes until fragrant.
3. Season and Finish:
   - Drizzle soy sauce and sesame oil over the stir-fried vegetables. Toss to coat evenly.
   - Sprinkle sesame seeds for garnish.
4. Serve:
   - Serve the Teriyaki Salmon over a bed of stir-fried vegetables.

Eggplant Parmesan:

Ingredients:

- 2 large eggplants, sliced into 1/2-inch rounds
- Salt, for sweating the eggplant
- 2 cups marinara sauce
- 2 cups mozzarella cheese, shredded
- 1 cup Parmesan cheese, grated
- 1 cup breadcrumbs (gluten-free if needed)
- 2 eggs, beaten
- 1/4 cup fresh basil, chopped

- 1/4 cup fresh parsley, chopped
- Olive oil, for brushing eggplant slices

Instructions:

1. Preheat Oven:
   - Preheat your oven to 375°F (190°C).
2. Prepare Eggplant:
   - Lay the eggplant slices on a paper towel and sprinkle with salt. Allow them to sit for 20-30 minutes to release excess moisture. Pat them dry with a paper towel.
3. Set Up Breading Station:
   - In one shallow dish, place the beaten eggs. In another dish, combine breadcrumbs with chopped fresh basil and parsley.
4. Bread the Eggplant:
   - Dip each eggplant slice into the beaten eggs, then coat with the breadcrumb mixture, pressing gently to adhere.
5. Cook Eggplant:
   - Heat olive oil in a large skillet over medium heat. Cook the breaded eggplant slices for 2-3 minutes on each side or until golden brown. Place them on a paper towel-lined plate to absorb excess oil.
6. Assemble Eggplant Parmesan:
   - In a baking dish, spread a thin layer of marinara sauce.
   - Arrange a layer of cooked eggplant slices on top.
   - Sprinkle it with mozzarella and Parmesan cheeses.
   - Repeat the layers, finishing with a layer of cheese on top.
7. Bake:
   - Bake in the preheated oven for 25-30 minutes or until the cheese is melted and bubbly and the eggplant is tender.
8. Garnish and Serve:
   - Garnish with additional fresh basil and parsley if desired.

   o Allow it to cool for a few minutes before serving.

Taco Salad Bowl:

Ingredients:

For the Taco Seasoned Meat:

- 1 pound ground beef or ground turkey
- 1 packet taco seasoning
- 1/2 cup water

For the Salad:

- 1 head iceberg lettuce, shredded
- 1 cup cherry tomatoes, halved
- 1 cup black beans, drained and rinsed
- 1 cup corn kernels (fresh, frozen, or canned)
- 1 cup shredded cheddar cheese
- 1 avocado, sliced
- 1/2 red onion, finely chopped

For the Dressing:

- 1/2 cup sour cream
- 2 tablespoons mayonnaise
- 1 tablespoon taco seasoning

Optional Toppings:

- Salsa
- Guacamole
- Fresh cilantro
- Lime wedges
- Tortilla strips or crushed tortilla chips

Instructions:

1. Cook Taco Seasoned Meat:

- In a skillet over medium heat, cook the ground meat until browned. Drain excess fat if needed.
   - Add taco seasoning and water. Simmer until the mixture thickens and is well-coated with seasoning.
2. Prepare Salad Ingredients:
   - In a large bowl, combine shredded lettuce, halved cherry tomatoes, black beans, corn, shredded cheddar cheese, avocado slices and chopped red onion.
3. Make the Dressing:
   - In a small bowl, whisk together sour cream, mayonnaise, and taco seasoning. Adjust seasoning to taste.
4. Assemble Taco Salad Bowl:
   - Spoon the taco seasoned meat over the salad mixture.
   - Drizzle the dressing over the top.
5. Add Optional Toppings:
   - Garnish with salsa, guacamole, fresh cilantro, lime wedges and tortilla strips or crushed tortilla chips if desired.
6. Toss and Serve:
   - Toss the salad until well coated with the dressing and toppings.
   - Serve immediately.

Gluten-Free Chicken Alfredo Pasta:

Ingredients:

- 8 oz gluten-free fettuccine pasta
- 1 pound boneless, skinless chicken breasts, cut into bite-sized pieces
- 2 tablespoons olive oil
- 3 cloves garlic, minced
- 1 cup heavy cream
- 1 cup grated Parmesan cheese

- Salt and black pepper to taste
- 1/2 teaspoon nutmeg (optional)
- Fresh parsley, chopped for garnish

Instructions:

1. Cook Gluten-Free Pasta:
   - Cook the gluten-free fettuccine pasta according to package instructions. Drain and set aside.
2. Cook Chicken:
   - Season chicken pieces with salt and pepper.
   - In a large skillet, heat olive oil over medium-high heat.
   - Add chicken and cook until browned and cooked through. Remove chicken from the skillet and set aside.
3. Prepare Alfredo Sauce:
   - In the same skillet, add minced garlic and sauté for about 1 minute.
   - Pour in the heavy cream, stirring continuously. Bring it to a simmer.
4. Add Parmesan and Seasonings:
   - Reduce heat to low. Gradually add grated Parmesan cheese, stirring constantly until the cheese is melted and the sauce is smooth.
   - Season with salt, black pepper and nutmeg (if using).
5. Combine Pasta and Chicken:
   - Add the cooked chicken back into the skillet with the Alfredo sauce.
   - Toss in the cooked gluten-free fettuccine pasta. Stir until the pasta and chicken are well coated with the sauce.
6. Garnish and Serve:
   - Garnish with fresh chopped parsley.
   - Serve the gluten-free chicken Alfredo pasta immediately.

Cauliflower Fried Rice:

Ingredients:

- 1 medium-sized cauliflower head, grated or riced
- 2 tablespoons sesame oil
- 2 cloves garlic, minced
- 1 cup mixed vegetables (e.g carrots, peas, corn, diced bell peppers)
- 2 green onions, chopped
- 2 eggs, beaten
- 3 tablespoons soy sauce or tamari (gluten-free)
- 1 teaspoon ginger, grated
- 1 tablespoon rice vinegar
- Salt and pepper to taste
- Optional: Cooked and diced chicken, shrimp or tofu for protein

Instructions:

1. Prepare Cauliflower Rice:
   - Grate the cauliflower head or use a food processor to create cauliflower rice.
2. Cook Vegetables:
   - Heat sesame oil in a large skillet or wok over medium heat.
   - Add minced garlic and cook for about 30 seconds.
   - Add mixed vegetables and sauté until they are tender yet still crisp.
3. Add Cauliflower Rice:
   - Push the vegetables to the side of the skillet, making space for the cauliflower rice.
   - Add the cauliflower rice and stir to combine with the vegetables.
4. Create Well for Eggs:
   - Push the cauliflower rice and vegetables to the sides, creating a well in the center.
   - Pour beaten eggs into the well and scramble. Allow them to set slightly before mixing with the rice and veggies.
5. Season and Flavor:

    ○ Stir in soy sauce or tamari, grated ginger and rice vinegar. Mix well.

    ○ Season with salt and pepper to taste.

6. Optional Protein:

    ○ If adding protein, such as chicken, shrimp or tofu, add it at this stage and cook until fully heated through.

7. Finish with Green Onions:

    ○ Add chopped green onions and stir to combine.

8. Serve:

    ○ Serve the cauliflower fried rice hot, optionally garnished with additional green onions.

Moroccan Chickpea Stew:

Ingredients:

- 2 tablespoons olive oil
- 1 large onion, finely chopped
- 3 cloves garlic, minced
- 1 teaspoon ground cumin
- 1 teaspoon ground coriander
- 1 teaspoon ground turmeric
- 1/2 teaspoon cinnamon
- 1/4 teaspoon cayenne pepper (adjust to taste)
- 1 can (15 oz) chickpeas, drained and rinsed
- 1 can (15 oz) diced tomatoes
- 1 large carrot, peeled and diced
- 1 sweet potato, peeled and diced
- 4 cups vegetable broth
- 1 cup green beans, trimmed and halved
- 1/2 cup dried apricots, chopped
- Zest and juice of 1 lemon

- Salt and pepper to taste
- Fresh cilantro, chopped, for garnish
- Cooked couscous or rice for serving

Instructions:

1. Sauté Aromatics:
   - In a large pot, heat olive oil over medium heat. Add chopped onion and sauté until softened.
2. Add Spices:
   - Stir in minced garlic, ground cumin, ground coriander, ground turmeric, cinnamon and cayenne pepper. Cook for an additional 1-2 minutes until fragrant.
3. Combine Chickpeas and Vegetables:
   - Add drained chickpeas, diced tomatoes, diced carrot and diced sweet potato to the pot. Mix well to coat the vegetables with the spices.
4. Pour in Vegetable Broth:
   - Pour in vegetable broth and bring the stew to a simmer.
5. Cook and Add More Ingredients:
   - Once simmering, add green beans and chopped dried apricots. Continue simmering until all the vegetables are tender approximately 15-20 minutes.
6. Season and Finish:
   - Stir in lemon zest and juice.
   - Season with salt and pepper to taste.
7. Garnish and Serve:
   - Garnish with fresh chopped cilantro.
   - Serve the Moroccan Chickpea Stew over cooked couscous or rice.

Lemon Herb Shrimp Skewers:

Ingredients:
- 1 pound large shrimp, peeled and deveined

- Zest and juice of 2 lemons
- 3 tablespoons olive oil
- 2 cloves garlic, minced
- 1 teaspoon dried oregano
- 1 teaspoon dried thyme
- 1 teaspoon paprika
- Salt and black pepper to taste
- Fresh parsley, chopped, for garnish
- Lemon wedges for serving

Instructions:

1. Marinate Shrimp:
   - In a bowl, whisk together lemon zest, lemon juice, olive oil, minced garlic, dried oregano, dried thyme, paprika, salt and black pepper.
   - Add the peeled and deveined shrimp to the marinade. Toss to coat. Allow the shrimp to marinate for at least 15-20 minutes.
2. Preheat Grill or Skillet:
   - Preheat your grill or skillet over medium-high heat.
3. Skewer Shrimp:
   - Thread the marinated shrimp on skewers. If using wooden skewers, make sure to soak them in water for about 15 minutes before threading to prevent burning.
4. Grill Shrimp:
   - Grill the shrimp skewers for 2-3 minutes per side or until they are opaque and have grill marks.
5. Garnish and Serve:
   - Sprinkle chopped fresh parsley over the grilled shrimp.
   - Serve the lemon herb shrimp skewers hot with lemon wedges on the side.

Gluten-Free BBQ Pulled Pork Sandwich:

Ingredients:

For the Pulled Pork:

- 2-3 pounds pork shoulder or pork butt
- 1 tablespoon smoked paprika
- 1 tablespoon garlic powder
- 1 tablespoon onion powder
- 1 tablespoon brown sugar

- 1 teaspoon salt
- 1/2 teaspoon black pepper
- 1 cup gluten-free barbecue sauce
- 1 cup chicken or vegetable broth

For the Gluten-Free Sandwich:

- Gluten-free hamburger buns or sandwich bread
- Coleslaw (store-bought or homemade)
- Pickles, sliced (optional)

Instructions:

1. **Prepare the Pork:**
   - In a small bowl, mix together smoked paprika, garlic powder, onion powder, brown sugar, salt and black pepper to create a dry rub.
   - Rub the dry rub all over the pork shoulder or pork butt, covering it evenly.
2. Slow Cook the Pork:
   - Place the seasoned pork in a slow cooker.
   - Pour the barbecue sauce and broth over the pork.
   - Cook on low for 8-10 hours or until the pork is tender and easily pulls apart.
3. Shred the Pork:
   - Once cooked, shred the pork using two forks. Mix the shredded pork with the cooking liquid to enhance flavor.
4. Assemble Sandwich:
   - Toast gluten-free hamburger buns or sandwich bread.
   - Place a generous amount of the pulled pork on the bottom half of each bun.
5. Add Toppings:
   - Top the pulled pork with coleslaw and sliced pickles if desired.
6. Serve:
   - Place the top half of the bun on the coleslaw to complete the sandwich.

Zucchini Noodles with Pesto:

Ingredients:

For the Pesto:

- 2 cups fresh basil leaves, packed
- 1/2 cup grated Parmesan cheese
- 1/2 cup pine nuts or walnuts

- 3 cloves garlic, peeled

- 1/2 cup extra virgin olive oil

- Salt and black pepper to taste

- Juice of 1 lemon (optional)

For the Zucchini Noodles:

- 4 medium-sized zucchini, spiralized

- 1 tablespoon olive oil

- Salt and black pepper to taste

- Grated Parmesan cheese for garnish (optional)

Instructions:

1. Make the Pesto:
   - In a food processor, combine fresh basil, grated Parmesan cheese, pine nuts or walnuts and peeled garlic cloves.
   - Pulse until coarsely chopped.
   - With the food processor running, gradually pour in the olive oil until the pesto reaches your desired consistency.
   - Season with salt and black pepper. Add lemon juice if desired for a citrusy kick.

2. Prepare Zucchini Noodles:
   - Spiralize the zucchini into noodle-like strands using a spiralizer.
   - Heat olive oil in a large skillet over medium heat.
   - Add the zucchini noodles to the skillet, sautéing for 2-3 minutes until they are just tender but still have a slight crunch.
   - Season with salt and black pepper.

3. Combine with Pesto:
   - Add the prepared pesto to the zucchini noodles in the skillet. Toss until the noodles are well coated with the pesto.

4. Serve:
   - Transfer the zucchini noodles with pesto to serving plates.
   - Optionally, garnish with additional grated Parmesan cheese.

Mediterranean Quinoa Salad:

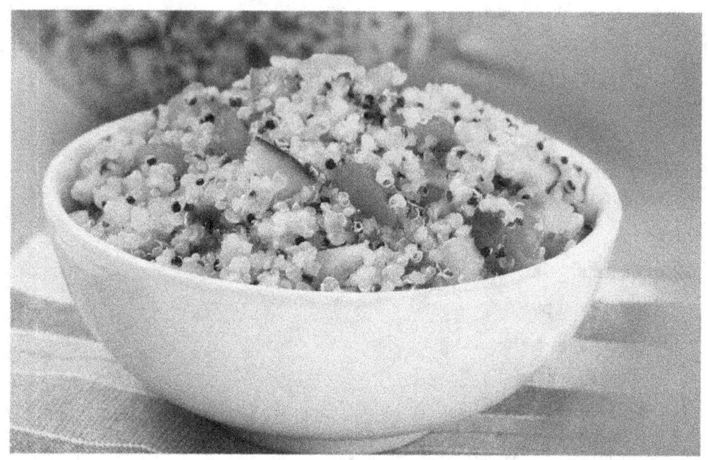

Ingredients:

- 1 cup quinoa, rinsed
- 2 cups water or vegetable broth
- 1 cup cherry tomatoes, halved
- 1 cucumber, diced
- 1/2 red onion, finely chopped
- 1/2 cup Kalamata olives, pitted and sliced
- 1/2 cup feta cheese, crumbled
- 1/4 cup fresh parsley, chopped
- 1/4 cup fresh mint, chopped

For the Dressing:

- 1/4 cup extra virgin olive oil
- 2 tablespoons red wine vinegar

- 1 teaspoon Dijon mustard
- 1 clove garlic, minced
- Salt and black pepper to taste

Instructions:

1. Cook Quinoa:
   - In a medium saucepan, combine quinoa and water or vegetable broth.
   - Bring to a boil, then reduce heat to low, cover, and simmer for 15-20 minutes or until quinoa is cooked and water is absorbed.
   - Fluff quinoa with a fork and let it cool.
2. Prepare Vegetables:
   - In a large bowl, combine cherry tomatoes, diced cucumber, chopped red onion, sliced Kalamata olives, crumbled feta cheese, fresh parsley and fresh mint.
3. Make the Dressing:
   - In a small bowl, whisk together extra virgin olive oil, red wine vinegar, Dijon mustard, minced garlic, salt and black pepper.
4. Combine Quinoa and Vegetables:
   - Add the cooked quinoa to the bowl of vegetables.
5. Drizzle with Dressing:
   - Pour the dressing over the quinoa and vegetables.
6. Toss Gently:
   - Gently toss the salad until all ingredients are well combined and coated with the dressing.
7. Chill and Serve:
   - Refrigerate the Mediterranean quinoa salad for at least 30 minutes before serving to allow the flavors to meld.

Caprese Salad with Balsamic Glaze:

Ingredients:

- 4 large tomatoes, sliced
- 1 pound fresh mozzarella cheese, sliced
- Fresh basil leaves
- Balsamic glaze
- Extra virgin olive oil
- Salt and black pepper to taste

Instructions:

1. Slice Tomatoes and Mozzarella:
   - Slice the tomatoes and fresh mozzarella into rounds of similar thickness.
2. Arrange on a Platter:
   - Arrange the tomato and mozzarella slices on a serving platter, alternating them for an appealing presentation.
3. Layer with Basil:
   - Place fresh basil leaves between the tomato and mozzarella slices. You can also tuck them underneath for a layered effect.
4. Season with Salt and Pepper:
   - Sprinkle salt and black pepper over the tomato and mozzarella slices to taste.
5. Drizzle with Olive Oil:
   - Drizzle extra virgin olive oil over the Caprese salad for added flavor.
6. Balsamic Glaze:
   - Generously drizzle balsamic glaze over the salad. The sweet and tangy glaze complements the freshness of the tomatoes and mozzarella.
7. Serve:
   - Serve the Caprese salad immediately as a refreshing appetizer or side dish.

Grilled Chicken Caesar Salad:

Ingredients:

For the Grilled Chicken:

- 2 boneless, skinless chicken breasts
- 2 tablespoons olive oil
- 1 teaspoon garlic powder
- 1 teaspoon dried oregano
- Salt and black pepper to taste

For the Caesar Dressing:

- 1/2 cup mayonnaise
- 1/4 cup grated Parmesan cheese
- 2 tablespoons Dijon mustard
- 2 cloves garlic, minced
- 2 tablespoons anchovy paste (optional)
- 1 tablespoon Worcestershire sauce
- Juice of 1 lemon
- Salt and black pepper to taste

For the Salad:

- Romaine lettuce, chopped
- Croutons (store-bought or homemade)
- Additional grated Parmesan cheese for garnish

Instructions:

1. Marinate and Grill Chicken:
   - In a bowl, combine olive oil, garlic powder, dried oregano, salt and black pepper.
   - Marinate the chicken breasts in this mixture for at least 30 minutes.
   - Grill the chicken breasts until fully cooked, approximately 6-8 minutes per side. Allow them to rest before slicing.
2. Prepare Caesar Dressing:
   - In a bowl, whisk together mayonnaise, grated Parmesan cheese, Dijon mustard, minced garlic, anchovy paste (if using), Worcestershire sauce, lemon juice, salt and black pepper. Adjust seasoning to taste.

3. Assemble Salad:
   - Chop the grilled chicken into slices.
   - In a large bowl, combine chopped Romaine lettuce with croutons.
   - Add the sliced grilled chicken to the salad.
4. Dress Salad:
   - Drizzle the Caesar dressing over the salad. Toss until all ingredients are well coated.
5. Garnish:
   - Garnish the Grilled Chicken Caesar Salad with additional grated Parmesan cheese.
6. Serve:
   - Serve the salad immediately as a hearty and satisfying meal.

Avocado and Black Bean Salad:

Ingredients:

- 1 can (15 oz) black beans, drained and rinsed
- 2 ripe avocados, diced
- 1 cup corn kernels (fresh, frozen or canned)
- 1 cup cherry tomatoes, halved
- 1/2 red onion, finely chopped
- 1/4 cup fresh cilantro, chopped
- Juice of 2 limes
- 2 tablespoons extra virgin olive oil
- Salt and black pepper to taste
- Optional: Red pepper flakes for heat

Instructions:

1. Prepare Ingredients:
   - Rinse and drain the black beans.
   - Dice the ripe avocados.

- If using fresh corn, cook it and allow it to cool. If using frozen or canned corn, make sure it's thawed or drained.

2. Combine Ingredients:
   - In a large bowl, combine black beans, diced avocados, corn kernels, halved cherry tomatoes, finely chopped red onion and chopped fresh cilantro.

3. Make the Dressing:
   - In a small bowl, whisk together lime juice, extra virgin olive oil, salt and black pepper. Adjust the seasoning to taste.
   - Optionally, add red pepper flakes for a hint of heat.

4. Toss and Coat:
   - Pour the dressing over the salad ingredients.
   - Gently toss until all ingredients are well coated with the dressing.

5. Chill and Serve:
   - Refrigerate the Avocado and Black Bean Salad for at least 15-20 minutes before serving to allow the flavors to meld.

Asian Sesame Ginger Salad:

Ingredients:

For the Salad:

- 6 cups mixed salad greens (e.g Romaine lettuce, spinach, arugula)
- 1 cup shredded red cabbage
- 1 cup shredded carrots
- 1 red bell pepper, thinly sliced
- 1 cucumber, julienned
- 1/2 cup edamame, cooked and shelled
- 1/4 cup chopped green onions
- 1/4 cup chopped cilantro

For the Sesame Ginger Dressing:

- 3 tablespoons soy sauce

- 2 tablespoons rice vinegar
- 1 tablespoon sesame oil
- 1 tablespoon olive oil
- 1 tablespoon honey or maple syrup
- 1 tablespoon freshly grated ginger
- 2 cloves garlic, minced
- 1 tablespoon sesame seeds (optional)
- Salt and black pepper to taste

Instructions:

1. Prepare Salad Ingredients:
   - In a large bowl, combine mixed salad greens, shredded red cabbage, shredded carrots, thinly sliced red bell pepper, julienned cucumber, edamame, chopped green onions and chopped cilantro.
2. Make Sesame Ginger Dressing:
   - In a small bowl, whisk together soy sauce, rice vinegar, sesame oil, olive oil, honey or maple syrup, freshly grated ginger, minced garlic, sesame seeds (if using), salt and black pepper.
3. Dress the Salad:
   - Drizzle the Sesame Ginger Dressing over the salad.
4. Toss Gently:
   - Gently toss the salad until all ingredients are well coated with the dressing.
5. Chill and Serve:
   - Refrigerate the Asian Sesame Ginger Salad for about 15 minutes before serving to allow the flavors to meld.

Roasted Vegetable Salad:

Ingredients:

For the Roasted Vegetables:

- 2 cups cherry tomatoes, halved

- 2 bell peppers, diced (assorted colors)
- 1 zucchini, sliced
- 1 yellow squash, sliced
- 1 red onion, sliced
- 2 tablespoons olive oil
- 1 teaspoon dried thyme
- 1 teaspoon dried rosemary
- Salt and black pepper to taste

For the Salad:

- Mixed salad greens (e.g arugula, spinach or your favorite greens)
- 1/2 cup feta cheese, crumbled
- 1/4 cup fresh basil, chopped
- Balsamic glaze for drizzling

Instructions:

1. Preheat Oven:
   - Preheat the oven to 400°F (200°C).
2. Prepare Vegetables:
   - In a large bowl, combine cherry tomatoes, diced bell peppers, sliced zucchini, sliced yellow squash and sliced red onion.
   - Drizzle olive oil over the vegetables and toss to coat.
   - Sprinkle dried thyme, dried rosemary, salt, and black pepper. Toss again to evenly distribute the seasonings.
3. Roast Vegetables:
   - Spread the seasoned vegetables on a baking sheet in a single layer.
   - Roast in the preheated oven for 20-25 minutes or until the vegetables are tender and slightly caramelized.
4. Assemble Salad:
   - In a large serving bowl, arrange mixed salad greens.
   - Top with the roasted vegetables.

5. Add Feta and Basil:

    ○ Sprinkle crumbled feta cheese over the roasted vegetables.

    ○ Add fresh chopped basil for a burst of flavor.

6. Drizzle with Balsamic Glaze:

    ○ Finish the salad by drizzling balsamic glaze over the top.

7. Serve:

    ○ Serve the Roasted Vegetable Salad as a delicious and hearty side dish or a light main course.

Spinach and Strawberry Salad:

Ingredients:

- 6 cups baby spinach leaves, washed and dried
- 1 pint strawberries, hulled and sliced
- 1/2 cup feta cheese, crumbled
- 1/4 cup red onion, thinly sliced
- 1/4 cup sliced almonds, toasted

For the Balsamic Vinaigrette:

- 3 tablespoons balsamic vinegar
- 1/4 cup extra virgin olive oil
- 1 teaspoon Dijon mustard
- 1 teaspoon honey or maple syrup
- Salt and black pepper to taste

Instructions:

1. Prepare Spinach and Strawberries:

    ○ In a large bowl, combine baby spinach leaves with sliced strawberries.

2. Add Feta, Red Onion, and Almonds:

    ○ Sprinkle crumbled feta cheese over the salad.

    ○ Add thinly sliced red onion and toasted sliced almonds for additional texture and flavor.

3. Make Balsamic Vinaigrette:
    - In a small bowl or jar, whisk together balsamic vinegar, extra virgin olive oil, Dijon mustard, honey or maple syrup, salt, and black pepper. Adjust the sweetness and acidity to your taste.
4. Dress the Salad:
    - Drizzle the Balsamic Vinaigrette over the spinach and strawberry mixture.
5. Toss Gently:
    - Gently toss the salad until all ingredients are well coated with the vinaigrette.
6. Serve:
    - Serve the Spinach and Strawberry Salad immediately

Chickpea and Feta Greek Salad:

Ingredients:

- 1 can (15 oz) chickpeas, drained and rinsed
- 1 cucumber, diced
- 1 cup cherry tomatoes, halved
- 1/2 red onion, finely chopped
- 1/2 cup Kalamata olives, pitted and sliced
- 1/2 cup crumbled feta cheese
- 1/4 cup fresh parsley, chopped

For the Greek Dressing:

- 1/4 cup extra virgin olive oil
- 2 tablespoons red wine vinegar
- 1 teaspoon dried oregano
- 1 clove garlic, minced
- Salt and black pepper to taste
- Optional: Lemon juice for added freshness

Instructions:

1. Prepare Chickpeas:
   - Drain and rinse chickpeas thoroughly.
2. Combine Ingredients:
   - In a large bowl, combine chickpeas, diced cucumber, halved cherry tomatoes, finely chopped red onion, sliced Kalamata olives, crumbled feta cheese and chopped fresh parsley.
3. Make Greek Dressing:
   - In a small bowl, whisk together extra virgin olive oil, red wine vinegar, dried oregano, minced garlic, salt and black pepper. Adjust seasoning to taste.
   - Optionally, add a splash of lemon juice for extra freshness.
4. Dress the Salad:
   - Pour the Greek dressing over the chickpea and feta mixture.
5. Toss Gently:
   - Gently toss the salad until all ingredients are well coated with the dressing.
6. Chill and Serve:
   - Refrigerate the Chickpea and Feta Greek Salad for about 15 minutes before serving to allow the flavors to meld.

Tuna Niçoise Salad:

Ingredients:
- 8 small red potatoes, halved
- 1 pound green beans, trimmed
- 4 large eggs
- 1 cup cherry tomatoes, halved
- 1/2 red onion, thinly sliced
- 1/2 cup Niçoise olives
- 2 cans (5 oz each) tuna in olive oil, drained
- Fresh parsley, chopped (for garnish)

For the Dijon Vinaigrette:

- 1/4 cup extra virgin olive oil
- 2 tablespoons red wine vinegar
- 1 tablespoon Dijon mustard
- 1 clove garlic, minced
- Salt and black pepper to taste

Instructions:

1. Boil Potatoes:
   - Boil halved red potatoes in salted water until fork-tender, approximately 12-15 minutes.
2. Blanch Green Beans:
   - Blanch the trimmed green beans in boiling water for 2-3 minutes, then transfer them to an ice bath to stop the cooking process.
3. Hard-Boil Eggs:
   - Hard-boil the eggs by placing them in a saucepan, covering them with water, bringing to a boil, then simmering for 8-10 minutes. Transfer eggs to an ice bath, peel and halve them.
4. Assemble Salad:
   - Arrange boiled potatoes, blanched green beans, halved cherry tomatoes, thinly sliced red onion, Niçoise olives and tuna on a serving platter.
5. Make Dijon Vinaigrette:
   - In a small bowl, whisk together extra virgin olive oil, red wine vinegar, Dijon mustard, minced garlic, salt and black pepper.
6. Drizzle Vinaigrette:
   - Drizzle the Dijon vinaigrette over the Tuna Nicoise Salad.
7. Garnish:
   - Garnish the salad with halved hard-boiled eggs and chopped fresh parsley.
8. Serve:
   - Serve the Tuna Niçoise Salad immediately.

Beet and Goat Cheese Salad:

Ingredients:

- 4 medium-sized beets, roasted and sliced
- 4 cups mixed salad greens (e.g arugula, baby spinach or mixed greens)
- 1/2 cup crumbled goat cheese
- 1/4 cup walnuts, toasted and chopped
- 2 tablespoons balsamic vinegar
- 3 tablespoons extra virgin olive oil
- 1 teaspoon honey or maple syrup
- Salt and black pepper to taste

Instructions:

1. Roast Beets:
   - Preheat the oven to 400°F (200°C).
   - Wrap each beet individually in aluminum foil and place them on a baking sheet.
   - Roast for about 45-60 minutes or until beets are fork-tender.
   - Allow the roasted beets to cool then peel and slice them.
2. Prepare Salad Greens:
   - In a large bowl, combine the mixed salad greens.
3. Add Beets, Goat Cheese and Walnuts:
   - Add the sliced roasted beets to the salad greens.
   - Sprinkle crumbled goat cheese and toasted, chopped walnuts over the salad.
4. Make Balsamic Vinaigrette:
   - In a small bowl, whisk together balsamic vinegar, extra virgin olive oil, honey or maple syrup, salt and black pepper.
5. Drizzle Vinaigrette:
   - Drizzle the balsamic vinaigrette over the beet and goat cheese salad.
6. Toss Gently:

- ○ Gently toss the salad until all ingredients are well coated with the vinaigrette.

7. Serve:

- ○ Serve the Beet and Goat Cheese Salad immediately as a vibrant and flavorful appetizer or side dish.

Cobb Salad with Avocado Ranch Dressing:

Ingredients:

For the Salad:

- 4 cups mixed salad greens (e.g Romaine lettuce, spinach)
- 1 cup cherry tomatoes, halved
- 2 cups cooked and diced chicken breast
- 4 hard-boiled eggs, sliced
- 1 cup crumbled blue cheese
- 1 avocado, diced
- 6 slices cooked bacon, crumbled

For the Avocado Ranch Dressing:

- 1 ripe avocado
- 1/2 cup buttermilk
- 1/4 cup mayonnaise
- 1 clove garlic, minced
- 2 tablespoons chopped fresh parsley
- 2 tablespoons chopped fresh chives
- 1 tablespoon white wine vinegar
- Salt and black pepper to taste

Instructions:

1. Prepare Salad Ingredients:

- ○ In a large bowl, arrange mixed salad greens as the base.

- Add halved cherry tomatoes, diced chicken breast, sliced hard-boiled eggs, crumbled blue cheese, diced avocado and crumbled bacon on top of the greens.

2. Make Avocado Ranch Dressing:
   - In a blender or food processor, combine ripe avocado, buttermilk, mayonnaise, minced garlic, chopped fresh parsley, chopped fresh chives, white wine vinegar, salt and black pepper.
   - Blend until smooth and creamy.
3. Dress the Salad:
   - Drizzle the Avocado Ranch Dressing over the Cobb Salad.
4. Serve:
   - Serve the Cobb Salad with Avocado Ranch Dressing immediately.

Soup Ideas:

Chicken and Vegetable Quinoa Soup:

Ingredients:

- 1 tablespoon olive oil
- 1 onion, diced
- 2 carrots, peeled and sliced
- 2 celery stalks, sliced
- 3 cloves garlic, minced
- 1 teaspoon dried thyme
- 1 teaspoon dried rosemary
- 1 teaspoon dried oregano
- 1 cup quinoa, rinsed
- 8 cups chicken broth
- 1 pound boneless, skinless chicken breasts, cooked and shredded
- 2 cups broccoli florets

- Salt and black pepper to taste
- Fresh parsley, chopped (for garnish)

Instructions:

1. Sauté Vegetables:
   - In a large pot, heat olive oil over medium heat.
   - Sauté diced onion, sliced carrots and sliced celery until softened.
2. Add Aromatics:
   - Stir in minced garlic, dried thyme, dried rosemary, and dried oregano. Cook for an additional 1-2 minutes until fragrant.
3. Add Quinoa and Broth:
   - Add rinsed quinoa to the pot and pour in chicken broth.
   - Bring the soup to a boil, then reduce heat to a simmer.
4. Cook Chicken:
   - In a separate pan, cook the chicken breasts until fully cooked. Shred the cooked chicken using forks.
5. Add Shredded Chicken and Broccoli:
   - Add the shredded cooked chicken and broccoli florets to the simmering soup.
6. Season:
   - Season the soup with salt and black pepper to taste. Adjust seasoning as needed.
7. Simmer:
   - Let the Chicken and Vegetable Quinoa Soup simmer for an additional 15-20 minutes or until the quinoa is cooked and the flavors meld together.
8. Garnish and Serve:
   - Garnish the soup with chopped fresh parsley before serving.

Tomato Basil Soup:

Ingredients:

- 2 tablespoons olive oil

- 1 onion, chopped

- 2 cloves garlic, minced

- 2 cans (28 oz each) whole peeled tomatoes

- 1 can (14 oz) crushed tomatoes

- 4 cups vegetable or chicken broth

- 1 teaspoon sugar

- 1/2 teaspoon dried oregano

- 1/2 teaspoon dried basil

- Salt and black pepper to taste

- 1/2 cup heavy cream (optional)

- Fresh basil leaves, for garnish

Instructions:

1. Sauté Onion and Garlic:

   - In a large pot, heat olive oil over medium heat. Add chopped onion and minced garlic, sauté until softened.

2. Add Tomatoes:

   - Pour in both cans of whole peeled tomatoes, including the juice. Break up the whole tomatoes using a spoon.
   - Add the crushed tomatoes.

3. Season and Simmer:

   - Stir in sugar, dried oregano, dried basil, salt and black pepper.
   - Pour in the vegetable or chicken broth. Bring the mixture to a simmer and let it cook for about 20-25 minutes.

4. Blend the Soup:

   - Use an immersion blender to carefully blend the soup until smooth. Alternatively, transfer the soup to a blender in batches, blend and return to the pot.

5. Optional Creamy Texture:

    ○ If desired, add heavy cream to the soup for a creamy texture. Stir well.

6. Adjust Seasoning:

    ○ Taste the soup and adjust the seasoning, adding more salt or pepper if needed.

7. Serve:

    ○ Ladle the Tomato Basil Soup into bowls.

    ○ Garnish each serving with fresh basil leaves.

Butternut Squash and Apple Soup:

Ingredients:

- 1 medium-sized butternut squash, peeled, seeded and diced
- 2 apples, peeled, cored and diced
- 1 onion, chopped
- 2 carrots, peeled and chopped
- 2 tablespoons olive oil
- 4 cups vegetable or chicken broth
- 1 teaspoon ground cinnamon
- 1/2 teaspoon ground nutmeg
- Salt and black pepper to taste
- 1 cup coconut milk or heavy cream
- Chopped fresh parsley or chives for garnish

Instructions:

1. Prepare Ingredients:

    ○ Peel, seed and dice the butternut squash.

    ○ Peel, core and dice the apples.

    ○ Chop the onion and carrots.

2. Sauté Vegetables:

    ○ In a large pot, heat olive oil over medium heat.

    ○ Sauté chopped onion and carrots until softened.

3. Add Squash and Apples:
   - Add diced butternut squash and apples to the pot. Stir well.
4. Season:
   - Season with ground cinnamon, ground nutmeg, salt and black pepper. Stir to coat the vegetables and apples with the spices.
5. Add Broth:
   - Pour in vegetable or chicken broth. Bring the mixture to a boil.
6. Simmer:
   - Reduce the heat to a simmer and cook for about 20-25 minutes or until the butternut squash is tender.
7. Blend the Soup:
   - Use an immersion blender to carefully blend the soup until smooth. Alternatively, transfer the soup to a blender in batches, blend and return to the pot.
8. Add Coconut Milk or Cream:
   - Stir in coconut milk or heavy cream to achieve the desired creaminess. Adjust the consistency and seasonings if needed.
9. Warm Through:
   - Warm the soup through, but do not bring it to a boil once the cream is added.
10. Serve:
- Ladle the Butternut Squash and Apple Soup into bowls.
- Garnish each serving with chopped fresh parsley

Lentil and Vegetable Soup:

Ingredients:
- 1 cup dried lentils, rinsed and drained
- 2 tablespoons olive oil
- 1 onion, chopped

- 2 carrots, peeled and diced
- 2 celery stalks, diced
- 3 cloves garlic, minced
- 1 teaspoon ground cumin
- 1 teaspoon ground coriander
- 1 teaspoon smoked paprika
- 1 can (14 oz) diced tomatoes
- 6 cups vegetable or chicken broth
- 2 bay leaves
- 1 cup green beans, trimmed and chopped
- 1 zucchini, diced
- Salt and black pepper to taste
- Fresh parsley, chopped (for garnish)

Instructions:

1. Prepare Lentils:
   - Rinse and drain the lentils.
2. Sauté Vegetables.
   - In a large pot, heat olive oil over medium heat.
   - Sauté chopped onion, diced carrots and diced celery until softened.
3. Add Garlic and Spices:
   - Add minced garlic, ground cumin, ground coriander and smoked paprika. Stir for about 1-2 minutes until the spices are fragrant.
4. Combine Tomatoes and Broth:
   - Pour in the diced tomatoes (with their juice) and vegetable or chicken broth.
5. Add Lentils and Bay Leaves:
   - Add the rinsed lentils and bay leaves to the pot. Stir well.
6. Simmer:
   - Bring the soup to a simmer and let it cook for about 25-30 minutes or until the lentils are tender.

7. Add Green Beans and Zucchini:
    ○ Add chopped green beans and diced zucchini to the pot. Cook for an additional 10-15 minutes or until the vegetables are tender.
8. Season:
    ○ Season the Lentil and Vegetable Soup with salt and black pepper to taste. Adjust the seasoning as needed.
9. Remove Bay Leaves:
    ○ Discard the bay leaves.
10. Serve:
    ○ Ladle the soup into bowls.
    ○ Garnish each serving with chopped fresh parsley.

Gluten-Free Minestrone Soup:

Ingredients:

- 2 tablespoons olive oil
- 1 onion, chopped
- 2 carrots, peeled and diced
- 2 celery stalks, diced
- 3 cloves garlic, minced
- 1 zucchini, diced
- 1 cup green beans, chopped
- 1 can (14 oz) diced tomatoes
- 1 can (15 oz) cannellini beans, drained and rinsed
- 1/2 cup gluten-free small pasta (e.g rice or corn pasta)
- 6 cups gluten-free vegetable broth
- 2 teaspoons dried oregano
- 2 teaspoons dried basil
- Salt and black pepper to taste
- 2 cups fresh spinach or kale, chopped

- Grated Parmesan cheese (optional for serving)

Instructions:

1. **Sauté Vegetables:**
   - In a large pot, heat olive oil over medium heat.
   - Sauté chopped onion, diced carrots, diced celery and minced garlic until softened.

2. Add Zucchini and Green Beans:
   - Add diced zucchini and chopped green beans to the pot. Cook for an additional 5 minutes.

3. Combine Tomatoes and Broth:
   - Pour in the diced tomatoes (with their juice), cannellini beans, gluten-free pasta and gluten-free vegetable broth.

4. Season:
   - Stir in dried oregano, dried basil, salt and black pepper to taste.

5. Simmer:
   - Bring the soup to a simmer and let it cook for about 15-20 minutes or until the vegetables and pasta are tender.

6. Add Spinach or Kale:
   - Stir in chopped fresh spinach or kale and cook until wilted.

7. Adjust Seasoning:
   - Taste the Gluten-Free Minestrone Soup and adjust the seasoning if needed.

8. Serve:
   - Ladle the soup into bowls.
   - Optionally, sprinkle each serving with grated Parmesan cheese.

Thai Coconut Chicken Soup (Tom Kha Gai):

Ingredients:

- 1 pound boneless, skinless chicken thighs, thinly sliced
- 4 cups chicken broth

- 1 can (13.5 oz) coconut milk
- 2 lemongrass stalks, bruised and cut into 3-inch pieces
- 4 kaffir lime leaves, torn into pieces
- 3 slices galangal or ginger, thinly sliced
- 2 tablespoons fish sauce
- 1 tablespoon soy sauce
- 1 tablespoon lime juice
- 1 tablespoon brown sugar
- 2 Thai bird chilies, sliced (adjust to taste)
- 1 cup mushrooms, sliced
- 1 medium tomato, cut into wedges
- Fresh cilantro leaves, for garnish
- Thinly sliced green onions, for garnish

Instructions:

1. Prepare Ingredients:
   - Thinly slice the chicken thighs.
   - Bruise the lemongrass stalks by pressing on them with the back of a knife and cut into 3-inch pieces.
   - Tear kaffir lime leaves into pieces.
   - Thinly slice galangal or ginger.
   - Slice Thai bird chilies, mushrooms and tomato.

2. Simmer Broth:
   - In a large pot, combine chicken broth, coconut milk, lemongrass, kaffir lime leaves and galangal or ginger.
   - Bring the mixture to a simmer over medium heat.

3. Add Chicken and Ingredients:
   - Add thinly sliced chicken thighs to the simmering broth.
   - Stir in fish sauce, soy sauce, lime juice and brown sugar.

4. Include Vegetables:

o Add sliced Thai bird chilies, mushrooms, and tomato wedges to the pot.

o Simmer until the chicken is cooked through and the vegetables are tender.

5. Remove Aromatics:

   o Remove lemongrass stalks, kaffir lime leaves and galangal or ginger slices from the soup.

6. Adjust Seasoning:

   o Taste the soup and adjust the seasoning if needed, adding more fish sauce, lime juice or sugar to achieve the desired balance of flavors.

7. Serve:

   o Ladle the Thai Coconut Chicken Soup into bowls.

   o Garnish with fresh cilantro leaves and thinly sliced green onions.

Broccoli and Cheddar Soup:

Ingredients:

- 4 cups broccoli florets, fresh or frozen
- 1 large onion, chopped
- 2 carrots, peeled and diced
- 3 cups vegetable or chicken broth
- 2 cups sharp cheddar cheese, shredded
- 1 cup milk
- 1/4 cup all-purpose flour
- 1/4 cup unsalted butter
- 3 cloves garlic, minced
- 1/2 teaspoon dried mustard
- Salt and black pepper to taste
- 1/4 teaspoon nutmeg (optional for added flavor)
- Croutons or additional shredded cheddar for garnish (optional)

Instructions:

1. Sauté Vegetables:

o   In a large pot, melt butter over medium heat. Add chopped onion, diced carrots and minced garlic. Sauté until the vegetables are softened.

2. Add Flour and Make Roux:

    o   Sprinkle flour over the sautéed vegetables and stir continuously to create a roux. Cook for 2-3 minutes to remove the raw flour taste.

3. Pour in Broth:

    o   Gradually pour in the vegetable or chicken broth, stirring constantly to avoid lumps.

4. Simmer:

    o   Add broccoli florets to the pot. Bring the mixture to a simmer and let it cook for about 15-20 minutes or until the broccoli is tender.

5. Blend Soup:

    o   Use an immersion blender to carefully blend the soup until smooth. Alternatively, transfer the soup to a blender in batches, blend and return to the pot.

6. Add Cheese and Milk:

    o   Stir in shredded cheddar cheese until melted.

    o   Pour in milk and continue stirring until well combined.

7. Season:

    o   Add dried mustard, salt, black pepper and nutmeg (if using). Adjust seasoning to taste.

8. Simmer and Serve:

    o   Let the Broccoli and Cheddar Soup simmer for an additional 5-10 minutes to meld the flavors.

    o   Serve the soup hot, optionally garnished with croutons or additional shredded cheddar.

Moroccan Chickpea Soup:

Ingredients:

- 1 tablespoon olive oil
- 1 onion, chopped
- 2 carrots, peeled and diced
- 2 celery stalks, diced
- 3 cloves garlic, minced
- 1 teaspoon ground cumin
- 1 teaspoon ground coriander
- 1 teaspoon smoked paprika
- 1/2 teaspoon ground cinnamon
- 1/4 teaspoon cayenne pepper (adjust to taste)
- 1 can (15 oz) chickpeas, drained and rinsed
- 1 can (14 oz) diced tomatoes
- 6 cups vegetable broth
- 1 cup red lentils, rinsed
- 1/4 cup chopped dried apricots
- Zest and juice of 1 lemon
- Salt and black pepper to taste
- Fresh cilantro, chopped (for garnish)
- Greek yogurt or coconut yogurt (optional, for serving)

Instructions:

1. Sauté Vegetables:
   - In a large pot, heat olive oil over medium heat. Add chopped onion, diced carrots, and diced celery. Sauté until the vegetables are softened.

2. Add Spices:
   - Stir in minced garlic, ground cumin, ground coriander, smoked paprika, ground cinnamon and cayenne pepper. Cook for 1-2 minutes until the spices are fragrant.

3. Combine Chickpeas and Tomatoes:

    ○ Add drained and rinsed chickpeas, diced tomatoes, and vegetable broth to the pot.

4. Include Lentils and Apricots:

    ○ Stir in rinsed red lentils and chopped dried apricots.

5. Simmer:

    ○ Bring the soup to a simmer and let it cook for about 20-25 minutes or until the lentils are tender.

6. Add Lemon Zest and Juice:

    ○ Add the zest and juice of one lemon to the soup. Stir well.

7. Season:

    ○ Season the Moroccan Chickpea Soup with salt and black pepper to taste. Adjust the seasoning if needed.

8. Serve:

    ○ Ladle the soup into bowls.

    ○ Garnish each serving with chopped fresh cilantro.

Creamy Potato Leek Soup:

Ingredients:

- 2 tablespoons unsalted butter
- 3 leeks, white and light green parts, sliced
- 3 large potatoes, peeled and diced
- 1 onion, chopped
- 2 cloves garlic, minced
- 6 cups vegetable or chicken broth
- 1 bay leaf
- 1 teaspoon dried thyme
- Salt and black pepper to taste
- 1 cup whole milk or half-and-half
- 1/2 cup heavy cream

- Chives, chopped (for garnish)

Instructions:

1. Sauté Vegetables:
   - In a large pot, melt butter over medium heat. Add sliced leeks, diced potatoes, chopped onion and minced garlic. Sauté until the vegetables are softened.
2. Add Broth and Seasonings:
   - Pour in vegetable or chicken broth.
   - Add a bay leaf, dried thyme, salt and black pepper to taste.
3. Simmer:
   - Bring the soup to a simmer and let it cook for about 20-25 minutes or until the potatoes are tender.
4. Remove Bay Leaf:
   - Discard the bay leaf from the soup.
5. Blend Soup:
   - Use an immersion blender to carefully blend the soup until smooth. Alternatively, transfer the soup to a blender in batches, blend and return to the pot.
6. Add Milk and Cream:
   - Stir in whole milk or half-and-half and heavy cream. Heat the soup through but do not boil.
7. Adjust Seasoning:
   - Taste the Creamy Potato Leek Soup and adjust the seasoning if needed.
8. Serve:
   - Ladle the soup into bowls.
   - Garnish each serving with chopped chives.

Mexican Chicken Tortilla Soup:

Ingredients:

- 1 tablespoon olive oil
- 1 onion, diced
- 2 cloves garlic, minced
- 1 jalapeño, seeded and finely chopped
- 1 bell pepper, diced
- 1 carrot, diced
- 1 teaspoon ground cumin
- 1 teaspoon chili powder
- 1 teaspoon smoked paprika
- 1 can (14 oz) diced tomatoes
- 4 cups chicken broth
- 1 cup corn kernels (fresh, frozen, or canned)
- 1 cup black beans, drained and rinsed
- 2 cups cooked chicken, shredded
- Salt and black pepper to taste
- Juice of 1 lime
- Fresh cilantro, chopped (for garnish)
- Avocado slices, for topping
- Tortilla strips or chips, for serving

Instructions:

1. Sauté Aromatics:
   - In a large pot, heat olive oil over medium heat. Add diced onion, minced garlic, chopped jalapeño, diced bell pepper and diced carrot. Sauté until vegetables are softened.
2. Add Spices:
   - Stir in ground cumin, chili powder, and smoked paprika. Cook for 1-2 minutes until the spices are fragrant.
3. Combine Tomatoes and Broth:

    o Add diced tomatoes (with their juice) and chicken broth to the pot. Bring the mixture to a simmer.

4. Include Corn, Black Beans, and Chicken:
   o   Stir in corn kernels, drained and rinsed black beans, and shredded cooked chicken.

5. Season:
   o   Season the Mexican Chicken Tortilla Soup with salt and black pepper to taste.

6. Simmer:
   o   Let the soup simmer for about 15-20 minutes to allow the flavors to meld.

7. Finish and Serve:
   o   Squeeze lime juice into the soup just before serving.
   o   Ladle the soup into bowls.
   o   Garnish with chopped fresh cilantro and top each serving with avocado slices.
   o   Serve with tortilla strips or chips on the side.

Italian Wedding Soup:

Ingredients:

For the Meatballs:

- 1/2 pound ground beef
- 1/2 pound ground pork
- 1/2 cup breadcrumbs
- 1/4 cup grated Parmesan cheese
- 1/4 cup chopped fresh parsley
- 1 egg
- 2 cloves garlic, minced
- Salt and black pepper to taste

For the Soup:

- 1 tablespoon olive oil
- 1 onion, diced
- 2 carrots, peeled and sliced
- 2 celery stalks, sliced
- 8 cups chicken broth
- 1 cup acini di pepe pasta or small pasta of choice
- 4 cups fresh spinach or escarole, chopped
- Salt and black pepper to taste
- Grated Parmesan cheese (for serving)

Instructions:

For the Meatballs:

1. Preheat Oven:
   - Preheat the oven to 400°F (200°C).
2. Prepare Meatball Mixture:
   - In a bowl, combine ground beef, ground pork, breadcrumbs, grated Parmesan cheese, chopped fresh parsley, egg, minced garlic, salt and black pepper.
   - Mix the ingredients until well combined.
3. Form Meatballs:
   - Shape the mixture into small meatballs, about 1 inch in diameter.
   - Place the meatballs on a baking sheet lined with parchment paper.
4. Bake Meatballs:
   - Bake in the preheated oven for 15-20 minutes or until the meatballs are cooked through and browned on the outside.

For the Soup:

1. Sauté Vegetables:
   - In a large pot, heat olive oil over medium heat. Sauté diced onion, sliced carrots, and sliced celery until softened.
2. Add Broth and Pasta:

- Pour in chicken broth. Bring the broth to a simmer.
- Add acini di pepe pasta or small pasta of your choice. Cook until the pasta is al dente.

3. Include Meatballs and Greens:
   - Add the baked meatballs to the simmering soup.
   - Stir in chopped fresh spinach or escarole.

4. Season:
   - Season the Italian Wedding Soup with salt and black pepper to taste.

5. Simmer:
   - Let the soup simmer for an additional 10-15 minutes to allow flavors to meld.

6. Serve:
   - Ladle the soup into bowls.
   - Optionally, sprinkle each serving with grated Parmesan cheese.

CHAPTER 5: SEAFOOD AND MEAT

Grilled Lemon Garlic Shrimp:

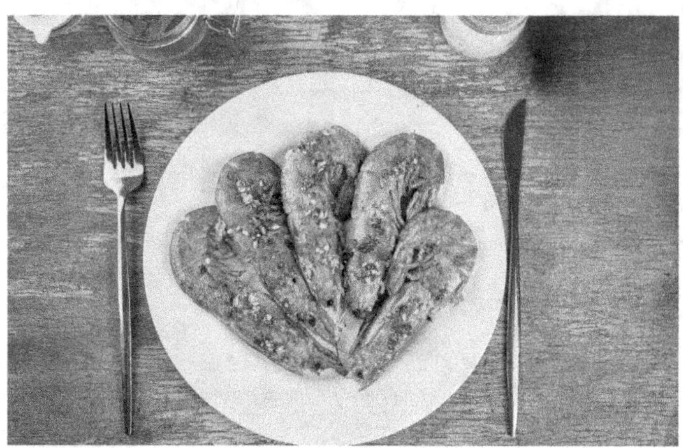

Ingredients:

- 1 pound large shrimp, peeled and deveined
- 3 tablespoons olive oil
- 3 cloves garlic, minced
- Zest of 1 lemon
- Juice of 1 lemon
- 1 teaspoon dried oregano
- 1/2 teaspoon paprika
- Salt and pepper to taste
- Skewers for grilling

Instructions:

1. Preheat your grill to medium-high heat.
2. In a bowl, mix together olive oil, minced garlic, lemon zest, lemon juice, oregano, paprika, salt, and pepper.

3. Thread the shrimp on skewers, ensuring they are evenly spaced.

4. Brush the shrimp skewers with the prepared lemon-garlic marinade, making sure to coat them thoroughly.

5. Place the skewers on the preheated grill and cook for 2-3 minutes per side or until the shrimp turn pink and opaque.

6. Baste the shrimp with any remaining marinade while grilling for added flavor.

7. Remove the shrimp skewers from the grill and serve hot, garnished with fresh lemon wedges and chopped parsley if desired!

Salmon with Dill Sauce:

Ingredients:

- 4 salmon fillets
- Salt and pepper to taste
- 2 tablespoons olive oil
- 1/4 cup chopped fresh dill
- 2 tablespoons Dijon mustard
- 2 tablespoons honey
- 2 tablespoons lemon juice
- 1/2 cup Greek yogurt

Instructions:

1. Preheat your oven to 400°F (200°C).

2. Season the salmon filets with salt and pepper on both sides.

3. Heat olive oil in an oven-safe skillet over medium-high heat.

4. Sear the salmon filets skin-side down for 2-3 minutes until golden brown.

5. Flip the filets and transfer the skillet to the preheated oven. Bake for 10-12 minutes or until the salmon flakes easily with a fork.

6. While the salmon is baking, prepare the dill sauce. In a bowl, mix together chopped dill, Dijon mustard, honey, lemon juice and Greek yogurt. Adjust seasoning to taste.

7. Once the salmon is done, remove it from the oven and drizzle the dill sauce over each filet.

8. Serve the salmon with additional dill sauce on the side, along with your favorite side dishes.

Gluten-Free Fish Tacos:

Ingredients:

For the Fish:

- 1 pound white fish filets (such as cod or tilapia)
- 1 cup gluten-free breadcrumbs
- 1/2 cup cornmeal
- 1 teaspoon paprika
- 1/2 teaspoon cumin
- Salt and pepper to taste
- 2 eggs, beaten
- Cooking oil for frying

For the Cabbage Slaw:

- 2 cups shredded cabbage
- 1/4 cup chopped fresh cilantro
- 1/4 cup mayonnaise
- 2 tablespoons lime juice
- Salt and pepper to taste

For Assembling Tacos:

- Gluten-free corn tortillas
- Avocado slices
- Lime wedges

Instructions:

1. In a shallow bowl, mix gluten-free breadcrumbs, cornmeal, paprika, cumin, salt, and pepper. Dip each fish filet into beaten eggs, then coat with the breadcrumb mixture.

2. Heat cooking oil in a pan over medium-high heat. Fry the breaded fish filets for 3-4 minutes per side or until golden brown and cooked through. Place on a paper towel-lined plate to drain excess oil.

3. In a separate bowl, combine shredded cabbage, chopped cilantro, mayonnaise, lime juice, salt and pepper. Mix well to create the cabbage slaw.

4. Warm the gluten-free corn tortillas according to package instructions.

5. Assemble the tacos by placing a piece of fried fish on each tortilla. Top with the cabbage slaw and avocado slices.

6. Serve the gluten-free fish tacos with lime wedges on the side.

Lemon Butter Garlic Scallops:

Ingredients:

- 1 pound large sea scallops, patted dry
- Salt and black pepper to taste
- 2 tablespoons olive oil
- 3 tablespoons unsalted butter
- 4 cloves garlic, minced
- Zest of 1 lemon
- Juice of 1 lemon
- 2 tablespoons chopped fresh parsley

Instructions:

1. Season the scallops with salt and black pepper on both sides.

2. Heat olive oil in a large skillet over medium-high heat.

3. Add the scallops to the skillet and sear for 2-3 minutes per side until golden brown and opaque in the center. Be careful not to overcrowd the pan; cook in batches if necessary.

4. Remove the scallops from the skillet and set them aside.

5. In the same skillet, melt butter over medium heat. Add minced garlic and sauté for 1-2 minutes until fragrant.

6. Stir in lemon zest and lemon juice, allowing the flavors to meld for an additional minute.

7. Return the seared scallops to the skillet, coating them with the lemon butter garlic sauce. Cook briefly to warm the scallops through.

8. Sprinkle chopped fresh parsley over the scallops for a burst of color and freshness.

9. Serve the lemon butter garlic scallops hot, drizzling any remaining sauce over them.

Crispy Baked Cod:

Ingredients:

- 4 cod filets
- 1 cup gluten-free breadcrumbs
- 1/4 cup grated Parmesan cheese
- 1 teaspoon garlic powder
- 1 teaspoon paprika
- 1/2 teaspoon dried thyme
- Salt and black pepper to taste
- 2 tablespoons olive oil
- Lemon wedges for serving

Instructions:

1. Preheat your oven to 400°F (200°C) and line a baking sheet with parchment paper.

2. In a shallow bowl, combine gluten-free breadcrumbs, grated Parmesan cheese, garlic powder, paprika, dried thyme, salt and black pepper. Mix well.

3. Pat the cod filets dry with paper towels. Brush each filet with olive oil, ensuring they are well-coated.

4. Dip each cod filet into the breadcrumb mixture, pressing the breadcrumbs onto the fish to adhere.

5. Place the coated cod filets on the prepared baking sheet.

6. Bake in the preheated oven for 12-15 minutes or until the cod is cooked through and the coating is golden and crispy.

7. Remove from the oven and let the crispy baked cod rest for a couple of minutes before serving.

8. Serve the crispy baked cod with lemon wedges on the side for a refreshing citrus touch.

Shrimp and Avocado Salad:

Ingredients:

- 1 pound large shrimp, peeled and deveined
- 2 tablespoons olive oil
- 1 teaspoon smoked paprika
- Salt and black pepper to taste
- 4 cups mixed salad greens
- 2 avocados, diced
- 1 cup cherry tomatoes, halved
- 1/4 cup red onion, thinly sliced
- 1/4 cup fresh cilantro, chopped

For the Dressing:

- 3 tablespoons olive oil
- 2 tablespoons lime juice
- 1 clove garlic, minced
- 1 teaspoon honey
- Salt and black pepper to taste

Instructions:

1. In a bowl, toss the shrimp with olive oil, smoked paprika, salt, and black pepper until well coated.

2. Heat a skillet over medium-high heat. Cook the seasoned shrimp for 2-3 minutes per side until they are opaque and cooked through. Set aside.

3. In a large salad bowl, combine the mixed salad greens, diced avocados, cherry tomatoes, sliced red onion and chopped cilantro.

4. In a small bowl, whisk together the dressing ingredients: olive oil, lime juice, minced garlic, honey, salt, and black pepper.

5. Add the cooked shrimp to the salad bowl.

6. Drizzle the dressing over the salad and shrimp. Gently toss to combine, ensuring everything is well coated.

7. Serve the shrimp and avocado salad immediately, garnished with extra cilantro if desired.

Sesame Ginger Glazed Salmon:

Ingredients:

- 4 salmon filets
- Salt and black pepper to taste
- 2 tablespoons sesame oil
- 3 tablespoons soy sauce
- 2 tablespoons honey
- 1 tablespoon rice vinegar
- 1 tablespoon fresh ginger, grated
- 2 cloves garlic, minced
- 1 tablespoon sesame seeds
- Sliced green onions for garnish

Instructions:

1. Preheat your oven to 400°F (200°C) and line a baking sheet with parchment paper.

2. Season the salmon filets with salt and black pepper on both sides.

3. In a small bowl, whisk together sesame oil, soy sauce, honey, rice vinegar, grated ginger and minced garlic to create the glaze.

4. Place the salmon filets on the prepared baking sheet.

5. Brush the glaze over each salmon filet, ensuring they are well coated. Reserve some glaze for later.

6. Sprinkle sesame seeds over the glazed salmon filets.

7. Bake in the preheated oven for 12-15 minutes or until the salmon is cooked through and flakes easily.

8. While the salmon is baking, heat the reserved glaze in a small saucepan over low heat until it thickens slightly.

9. Once the salmon is done, drizzle the thickened glaze over the filets.

10. Garnish with sliced green onions and serve the Sesame Ginger Glazed Salmon hot.

Gluten-Free Seafood Paella:

Ingredients:

- 1 cup gluten-free paella rice
- 1 pound mixed seafood (shrimp, mussels, calamari etc.)
- 2 tablespoons olive oil
- 1 onion, finely chopped
- 2 cloves garlic, minced
- 1 red bell pepper, diced
- 1 yellow bell pepper, diced
- 1 teaspoon smoked paprika
- 1/2 teaspoon saffron threads
- 2 cups gluten-free vegetable or fish broth
- 1 cup diced tomatoes (fresh or canned)
- Salt and black pepper to taste
- Lemon wedges for serving
- Fresh parsley, chopped for garnish

Instructions:

1. In a small bowl, soak the saffron threads in a couple of tablespoons of warm water.
2. Heat olive oil in a large paella pan or a wide, shallow skillet over medium heat.
3. Add chopped onion and cook until softened. Add minced garlic and cook for an additional minute.
4. Stir in diced red and yellow bell peppers, cooking until they start to soften.
5. Add gluten-free paella rice to the pan, stirring to coat the rice with the vegetable mixture.
6. Sprinkle smoked paprika over the rice and continue to cook for 1-2 minutes to enhance the flavors.
7. Pour in the saffron-infused water along with the saffron threads. Stir well.
8. Add diced tomatoes and continue to cook for another 2-3 minutes.
9. Pour in the gluten-free vegetable or fish broth. Bring the mixture to a simmer.
10. Arrange the mixed seafood over the rice, pressing them slightly into the mixture. Season with salt and black pepper to taste.
11. Cover the pan and let it simmer on low heat for about 20-25 minutes or until the rice is cooked and the seafood is tender.
12. If needed, you can uncover the pan towards the end to allow the bottom to crisp up slightly.
13. Garnish the gluten-free seafood paella with chopped fresh parsley and serve with lemon wedges on the side.

Coconut Curry Shrimp:

Ingredients:

- 1 pound large shrimp, peeled and deveined
- 2 tablespoons coconut oil
- 1 onion, finely chopped
- 3 cloves garlic, minced
- 1 tablespoon fresh ginger, grated

- 2 tablespoons red curry paste
- 1 can (14 oz) coconut milk
- 1 tablespoon soy sauce
- 1 tablespoon fish sauce
- 1 tablespoon brown sugar
- 1 red bell pepper, thinly sliced
- 1 cup snow peas, trimmed
- Fresh cilantro, chopped, for garnish
- Cooked rice for serving

Instructions:

1. Heat coconut oil in a large skillet over medium heat.
2. Add chopped onion, minced garlic, and grated ginger to the skillet. Sauté until the onion is softened.
3. Stir in red curry paste and cook for an additional 1-2 minutes to release the flavors.
4. Add the peeled and deveined shrimp to the skillet, cooking until they start to turn pink.
5. Pour in the coconut milk, soy sauce, fish sauce, and brown sugar. Stir to combine and let it simmer for 5-7 minutes to allow the flavors to meld.
6. Add thinly sliced red bell pepper and trimmed snow peas to the skillet. Cook until the vegetables are tender-crisp and the shrimp are fully cooked.
7. Adjust seasoning to taste, adding more soy sauce or fish sauce if needed.
8. Serve the coconut curry shrimp over cooked rice.
9. Garnish with chopped fresh cilantro.

Grilled Teriyaki Tuna Steaks:

Ingredients:

- 4 tuna steaks
- 1/2 cup soy sauce
- 1/4 cup mirin (sweet rice wine)

- 2 tablespoons honey
- 1 tablespoon sesame oil
- 2 cloves garlic, minced
- 1 tablespoon fresh ginger, grated
- 2 green onions, thinly sliced (for garnish)
- Sesame seeds (for garnish)
- Lemon wedges (for serving)

Instructions:

1. In a bowl, whisk together soy sauce, mirin, honey, sesame oil, minced garlic, and grated ginger to create the teriyaki marinade.
2. Place the tuna steaks in a shallow dish and pour half of the teriyaki marinade over them. Allow the tuna to marinate for at least 30 minutes, turning the steaks to coat evenly.
3. Preheat your grill to medium-high heat.
4. Remove the tuna steaks from the marinade and discard the used marinade.
5. Grill the tuna steaks for 2-3 minutes per side or until the desired level of doneness is reached. For medium-rare, aim for a slightly pink center.
6. While grilling, baste the tuna with the remaining teriyaki marinade for added flavor.
7. Once the tuna steaks are done, remove them from the grill and let them rest for a couple of minutes.
8. Garnish the grilled teriyaki tuna steaks with sliced green onions and sesame seeds.
9. Serve hot with lemon wedges on the side.

Lobster and Avocado Salad:

Ingredients:

For the Salad:

- 2 lobster tails, cooked and chopped
- 2 avocados, diced

- 1 cup cherry tomatoes, halved
- 1/4 cup red onion, finely chopped
- Mixed salad greens (lettuce, arugula or spinach)

For the Dressing:

- 3 tablespoons olive oil
- 2 tablespoons lemon juice
- 1 tablespoon Dijon mustard
- 1 clove garlic, minced
- Salt and black pepper to taste

Instructions:

1. In a large bowl, combine chopped lobster tails, diced avocados, halved cherry tomatoes and finely chopped red onion.
2. In a small bowl, whisk together olive oil, lemon juice, Dijon mustard, minced garlic, salt, and black pepper to create the dressing.
3. Pour the dressing over the lobster and avocado mixture. Gently toss to coat everything evenly.
4. Arrange a bed of mixed salad greens on serving plates.
5. Spoon the lobster and avocado mixture over the bed of greens.
6. Optionally, garnish with additional lemon wedges and fresh herbs such as parsley or chives.
7. Serve your Lobster and Avocado Salad immediately.

Meat Ideas:

Rosemary Garlic Roast Chicken:

Ingredients:

- 1 whole chicken (about 4-5 pounds)
- Salt and black pepper to taste
- 4 cloves garlic, minced

- 2 tablespoons fresh rosemary, chopped
- 2 tablespoons olive oil
- 1 lemon, halved
- 1 onion, quartered
- 2 carrots, peeled and cut into chunks
- 2 potatoes, peeled and cut into chunks

Instructions:

1. Preheat your oven to 425°F (220°C).
2. Rinse the whole chicken under cold water and pat it dry with paper towels.
3. Season the chicken inside and out with salt and black pepper.
4. In a small bowl, mix minced garlic, chopped fresh rosemary and olive oil to create a paste.
5. Rub the rosemary and garlic paste all over the outside of the chicken ensuring it is well-coated.
6. Place the lemon halves inside the chicken cavity for added flavor.
7. In a roasting pan, arrange the quartered onion, carrot chunks and potato chunks.
8. Place the seasoned chicken on top of the vegetables in the roasting pan.
9. Roast the chicken in the preheated oven for about 1 hour and 15 minutes or until the internal temperature reaches 165°F (74°C) and the skin is golden and crispy.
10. Baste the chicken with pan juices every 20-30 minutes to keep it moist.
11. Once done, remove the chicken from the oven and let it rest for 10-15 minutes before carving.
12. Serve the Rosemary Garlic Roast Chicken with the roasted vegetables.

Gluten-Free Meatball Subs:

Ingredients:

For the Meatballs:

- 1 pound ground beef
- 1/2 cup gluten-free breadcrumbs

- 1/4 cup grated Parmesan cheese
- 1 egg
- 2 cloves garlic, minced
- 1 teaspoon dried oregano
- Salt and black pepper to taste

For the Marinara Sauce:

- 2 cups gluten-free marinara sauce (store-bought or homemade)

For Assembling:

- Gluten-free sub rolls
- Mozzarella cheese, shredded
- Fresh basil leaves, chopped (optional)

Instructions:

1. Preheat your oven to 375°F (190°C).
2. In a bowl, combine ground beef, gluten-free breadcrumbs, grated Parmesan cheese, egg, minced garlic, dried oregano, salt and black pepper. Mix until well combined.
3. Shape the mixture into meatballs, about 1 to 1.5 inches in diameter.
4. Place the meatballs on a baking sheet lined with parchment paper.
5. Bake the meatballs in the preheated oven for 20-25 minutes or until they are cooked through and browned on the outside.
6. While the meatballs are baking, heat the gluten-free marinara sauce in a saucepan over medium heat.
7. Once the meatballs are done, add them to the marinara sauce, ensuring they are well-coated.
8. Slice the gluten-free sub rolls and place the meatballs with marinara sauce inside each roll.
9. Sprinkle shredded mozzarella cheese on top of the meatballs.
10. Broil the meatball subs in the oven for 3-5 minutes or until the cheese is melted and bubbly.

11. Optionally, sprinkle chopped fresh basil on top for added freshness.

12. Serve your Gluten-Free Meatball Subs hot and enjoy.

Balsamic Glazed Pork Chops:

Ingredients:

- 4 bone-in pork chops
- Salt and black pepper to taste
- 2 tablespoons olive oil
- 1/2 cup balsamic vinegar
- 1/4 cup honey
- 2 cloves garlic, minced
- 1 teaspoon dried rosemary (or 1 tablespoon fresh, chopped)
- 1 tablespoon Dijon mustard

Instructions:

1. Preheat your oven to 375°F (190°C).

2. Season the pork chops with salt and black pepper on both sides.

3. In an oven-safe skillet, heat olive oil over medium-high heat.

4. Sear the pork chops for 2-3 minutes per side until golden brown.

5. In a bowl, whisk together balsamic vinegar, honey, minced garlic, dried rosemary, and Dijon mustard.

6. Pour the balsamic glaze over the seared pork chops, ensuring they are well-coated.

7. Transfer the skillet to the preheated oven and bake for 15-20 minutes or until the internal temperature of the pork reaches 145°F (63°C).

8. While baking, baste the pork chops with the glaze from the skillet a couple of times.

9. Once done, remove the skillet from the oven and let the pork chops rest for a few minutes.

10. Serve the Balsamic Glazed Pork Chops hot, drizzling extra glaze over the top if desired.

Beef Stir-Fry with Vegetables:

Ingredients:

For the Beef Marinade:

- 1 pound flank steak, thinly sliced
- 2 tablespoons soy sauce
- 1 tablespoon oyster sauce
- 1 tablespoon cornstarch
- 1 teaspoon sesame oil
- 1 teaspoon sugar
- 1/2 teaspoon black pepper

For the Stir-Fry:

- 2 tablespoons vegetable oil
- 3 cups mixed vegetables (broccoli florets, bell peppers, carrots, snap peas etc.)
- 3 cloves garlic, minced
- 1 tablespoon fresh ginger, grated
- 1/4 cup soy sauce
- 2 tablespoons oyster sauce
- 1 tablespoon hoisin sauce
- 1 tablespoon rice vinegar
- 1 teaspoon sugar
- Cooked rice for serving

Instructions:

1. In a bowl, combine thinly sliced flank steak with soy sauce, oyster sauce, cornstarch, sesame oil, sugar, and black pepper. Let it marinate for at least 15-20 minutes.

2. Heat vegetable oil in a wok or large skillet over high heat.

3. Add the marinated beef to the hot pan, spreading it out to ensure even cooking. Stir-fry for 2-3 minutes until the beef is browned and cooked through. Remove the beef from the pan and set it aside.

4. In the same pan, add a bit more oil if needed. Add minced garlic and grated ginger, stir-frying for about 30 seconds until fragrant.

5. Add mixed vegetables to the pan. Stir-fry for 3-4 minutes until the vegetables are tender-crisp.

6. In a small bowl, mix together soy sauce, oyster sauce, hoisin sauce, rice vinegar and sugar.

7. Pour the sauce over the vegetables and stir to combine.

8. Add the cooked beef back to the pan, tossing everything together until well coated and heated through.

9. Serve the beef stir-fry over cooked rice.

Stuffed Bell Peppers with Ground Turkey:

Ingredients:

- 4 large bell peppers, halved and seeds removed
- 1 pound ground turkey
- 1 cup cooked quinoa or rice
- 1 cup black beans, drained and rinsed
- 1 cup corn kernels (fresh, frozen, or canned)
- 1 cup diced tomatoes
- 1/2 cup onion, finely chopped
- 2 cloves garlic, minced
- 1 teaspoon ground cumin
- 1 teaspoon chili powder
- Salt and black pepper to taste
- 1 cup shredded cheese (cheddar, Monterey Jack or a blend)
- Fresh cilantro, chopped, for garnish
- Sour cream or Greek yogurt for serving (optional)

Instructions:

1. Preheat your oven to 375°F (190°C).

2. Place the halved bell peppers in a baking dish, cut side up.

3. In a skillet over medium heat, cook the ground turkey until browned. Drain any excess fat.

4. Add chopped onion and minced garlic to the skillet with the cooked turkey. Cook for an additional 2-3 minutes until the onion is softened.

5. Stir in cooked quinoa or rice, black beans, corn, diced tomatoes, ground cumin, chili powder, salt, and black pepper. Mix well and cook for another 5 minutes.

6. Spoon the turkey and vegetable mixture into each bell pepper half, pressing it down gently.

7. Top each stuffed pepper with shredded cheese.

8. Cover the baking dish with foil and bake in the preheated oven for 25-30 minutes or until the peppers are tender.

9. Remove the foil and broil for an additional 2-3 minutes until the cheese is melted and bubbly.

10. Garnish with chopped cilantro.

11. Serve the Stuffed Bell Peppers with Ground Turkey hot, optionally with a dollop of sour cream or Greek yogurt.

Herb-Crusted Rack of Lamb:

Ingredients:

- 1 rack of lamb (about 1.5 to 2 pounds), frenched
- Salt and black pepper to taste
- 2 tablespoons Dijon mustard
- 2 tablespoons olive oil

For the Herb Crust:

- 1 cup fresh breadcrumbs
- 2 tablespoons fresh parsley, chopped
- 1 tablespoon fresh rosemary, chopped
- 1 tablespoon fresh thyme leaves

- 2 cloves garlic, minced

- Salt and black pepper to taste

Instructions:

1. Preheat your oven to 400°F (200°C).

2. Season the rack of lamb with salt and black pepper.

3. In a small bowl, mix Dijon mustard and olive oil. Brush the mustard mixture evenly over the lamb.

4. In another bowl, combine fresh breadcrumbs, chopped parsley, chopped rosemary, thyme leaves, minced garlic, salt and black pepper to create the herb crust.

5. Press the herb crust mixture onto the mustard-coated lamb, ensuring an even and thick coating.

6. Heat a skillet over medium-high heat. Sear the rack of lamb on all sides for 2-3 minutes until browned.

7. Transfer the seared lamb to a roasting pan or baking sheet.

8. Roast in the preheated oven for 20-25 minutes for medium-rare or adjust the cooking time based on your preferred doneness.

9. Allow the lamb to rest for 10 minutes before slicing.

10. Slice between the bones to serve individual chops.

Gluten-Free Spaghetti Bolognese:

Ingredients:

- 1 pound gluten-free spaghetti

- 1 tablespoon olive oil

- 1 onion, finely chopped

- 2 carrots, peeled and diced

- 2 celery stalks, diced

- 3 cloves garlic, minced

- 1 pound ground beef or ground turkey

- 1 can (14 oz) crushed tomatoes

- 1/2 cup red wine (optional)
- 1 teaspoon dried oregano
- 1 teaspoon dried basil
- Salt and black pepper to taste
- 1/4 teaspoon red pepper flakes (optional)
- Fresh basil or parsley for garnish
- Grated Parmesan cheese (optional)

Instructions:

1. Cook the gluten-free spaghetti according to the package instructions. Drain and set aside.
2. In a large skillet, heat olive oil over medium heat. Add chopped onion, diced carrots, and diced celery. Cook until the vegetables are softened.
3. Add minced garlic to the skillet and sauté for another 1-2 minutes until fragrant.
4. Push the vegetables to the side of the skillet and add ground beef or turkey. Cook until browned, breaking it up with a spoon as it cooks.
5. Pour in crushed tomatoes and red wine (if using). Stir to combine.
6. Season the sauce with dried oregano, dried basil, salt, black pepper and red pepper flakes (if using). Mix well.
7. Simmer the Bolognese sauce for at least 20-30 minutes to allow the flavors to meld. If it gets too thick, you can add a bit of water.
8. Taste and adjust the seasoning as needed.
9. Serve the gluten-free spaghetti topped with the Bolognese sauce.

Chicken Piccata:

Ingredients:

- 4 boneless, skinless chicken breasts
- Salt and black pepper to taste
- 1/2 cup gluten-free all-purpose flour
- 2 tablespoons olive oil

- 3 tablespoons unsalted butter, divided
- 1/2 cup chicken broth
- 1/4 cup fresh lemon juice
- 1/4 cup capers, drained
- 2 tablespoons fresh parsley, chopped
- Lemon slices for garnish (optional)

Instructions:

1. Season the chicken breasts with salt and black pepper.
2. Dredge the chicken breasts in gluten-free all-purpose flour, shaking off any excess.
3. In a large skillet, heat olive oil and 2 tablespoons of butter over medium-high heat.
4. Add the chicken breasts to the skillet and cook for 3-4 minutes per side or until golden brown and cooked through. Remove the chicken from the skillet and set it aside.
5. In the same skillet, add chicken broth, fresh lemon juice, and capers. Bring the mixture to a simmer, scraping the bottom of the pan to incorporate any browned bits.
6. Stir in the remaining tablespoon of butter and chopped fresh parsley. Simmer for an additional 2-3 minutes to thicken the sauce slightly.
7. Return the cooked chicken to the skillet, coating it with the lemon-caper sauce. Cook for an additional 2 minutes to heat through.
8. Serve the Chicken Piccata hot, garnished with lemon slices if desired.

BBQ Pulled Pork:

Ingredients:

- 3-4 pounds pork shoulder (or pork butt)
- Salt and black pepper to taste
- 1 tablespoon vegetable oil
- 1 large onion, finely chopped
- 3 cloves garlic, minced
- 1 cup barbecue sauce

- 1/2 cup apple cider vinegar
- 1/4 cup brown sugar
- 1 tablespoon Dijon mustard
- 1 teaspoon smoked paprika
- 1 teaspoon cumin
- 1/2 teaspoon cayenne pepper (optional)
- 1 cup chicken or vegetable broth
- Hamburger buns or rolls for serving
- Coleslaw for topping (optional)

Instructions:

1. Season the pork shoulder with salt and black pepper.
2. In a large skillet or Dutch oven, heat vegetable oil over medium-high heat. Sear the pork shoulder on all sides until browned.
3. Remove the pork from the skillet and set it aside.
4. In the same skillet, add chopped onion and minced garlic. Sauté until the onion is softened.
5. Add barbecue sauce, apple cider vinegar, brown sugar, Dijon mustard, smoked paprika, cumin and cayenne pepper (if using) to the skillet. Stir to combine.
6. Place the seared pork back into the skillet, coating it with the barbecue sauce mixture.
7. Pour in the chicken or vegetable broth, ensuring the pork is partially submerged.
8. Cover the skillet or Dutch oven and transfer it to a preheated oven at 325°F (163°C).
9. Roast for 3-4 hours or until the pork is tender and easily shreds with a fork.
10. Remove the pork from the oven and shred it using two forks.
11. Stir the shredded pork into the barbecue sauce mixture, ensuring it's well coated.
12. Serve the BBQ Pulled Pork on hamburger buns or rolls, topped with coleslaw if desired.

Homemade Gluten-Free Meatloaf:

Ingredients:

For the Meatloaf:

- 1 1/2 pounds ground beef (or a mixture of beef and pork)
- 1 cup gluten-free breadcrumbs
- 1/2 cup milk (dairy or non-dairy alternative)

- 1/4 cup ketchup

- 1 large egg

- 1 onion, finely chopped

- 2 cloves garlic, minced

- 1 teaspoon Worcestershire sauce

- 1 teaspoon dried thyme

- 1 teaspoon dried oregano

- Salt and black pepper to taste

For the Glaze:

- 1/4 cup ketchup

- 1 tablespoon brown sugar

- 1 tablespoon apple cider vinegar

Instructions:

1. Preheat your oven to 350°F (175°C).

2. In a large mixing bowl, combine ground beef, gluten-free breadcrumbs, milk, ketchup, egg, chopped onion, minced garlic, Worcestershire sauce, dried thyme, dried oregano, salt and black pepper. Mix until well combined.

3. Transfer the meat mixture to a greased or parchment-lined loaf pan, shaping it into a loaf.

4. In a small bowl, mix together ketchup, brown sugar, and apple cider vinegar to create the glaze.

5. Spread the glaze evenly over the top of the meatloaf.

6. Bake in the preheated oven for 1 to 1.5 hours or until the internal temperature reaches 160°F (71°C).

7. Allow the meatloaf to rest for 10 minutes before slicing.

8. Slice and serve the Homemade Gluten-Free Meatloaf with your favorite side dishes.

Tandoori Chicken Skewers:

Ingredients:
For the Marinade:
- 1 cup plain yogurt
- 2 tablespoons olive oil
- 2 tablespoons Tandoori spice blend
- 1 tablespoon ginger, grated
- 1 tablespoon garlic, minced
- 1 teaspoon ground cumin
- 1 teaspoon ground coriander
- 1 teaspoon smoked paprika
- 1 teaspoon turmeric
- 1 teaspoon chili powder (adjust to taste)
- Salt and black pepper to taste
- Juice of 1 lemon

For the Chicken Skewers:
- 1.5 to 2 pounds boneless, skinless chicken thighs, cut into bite-sized pieces
- Wooden or metal skewers, soaked if using wooden ones

Instructions:
1. In a large bowl, combine all the marinade ingredients: yogurt, olive oil, Tandoori spice blend, grated ginger, minced garlic, ground cumin, ground coriander, smoked paprika, turmeric, chili powder, salt, black pepper and lemon juice. Mix well.
2. Add the bite-sized chicken pieces to the marinade, ensuring they are well-coated. Cover the bowl and refrigerate for at least 2 hours or preferably overnight, to allow the flavors to infuse.
3. Preheat your grill or grill pan to medium-high heat.
4. Thread the marinated chicken pieces onto skewers.
5. Grill the Tandoori chicken skewers for about 10-15 minutes, turning occasionally, until the chicken is fully cooked and has a nice char.
6. Optionally, baste the chicken with extra marinade while grilling for added flavor.
7. Serve the Tandoori Chicken Skewers hot, garnished with chopped cilantro and accompanied by your favorite dipping sauce or raita.

CHAPTER 6: VEGETARIAN AND VEGAN

Eggplant Parmesan:

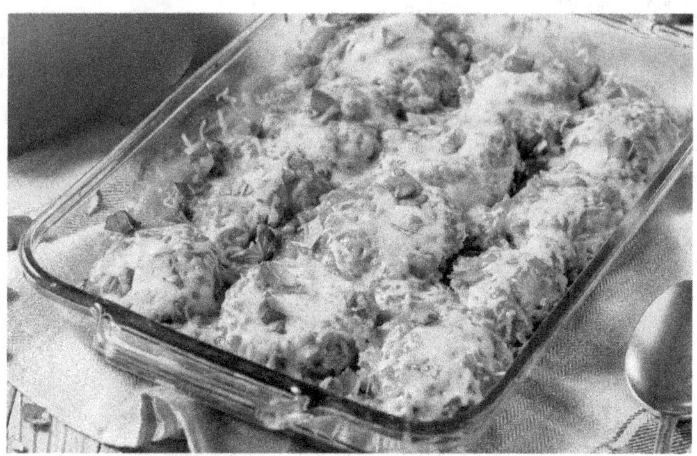

Ingredients:

- 2 large eggplants, sliced into 1/2-inch rounds
- Salt for sweating the eggplant
- 2 cups gluten-free breadcrumbs
- 1 cup grated Parmesan cheese
- 3 large eggs, beaten
- 2 cups marinara sauce (store-bought or homemade)
- 2 cups shredded mozzarella cheese
- Fresh basil or parsley, chopped for garnish

Instructions:

Preheat your oven to 375°F (190°C).

Place the eggplant slices in a colander and sprinkle each slice with salt. Let them sit for about 30 minutes to draw out excess moisture. Rinse the salt off and pat the slices dry with paper towels.

In a shallow bowl, combine gluten-free breadcrumbs and grated Parmesan cheese.

Dip each eggplant slice into the beaten eggs, allowing excess to drip off, and then coat with the breadcrumb mixture.

Place the coated eggplant slices on a baking sheet lined with parchment paper.

Bake the eggplant in the preheated oven for about 15-20 minutes or until they are golden and tender. Flip the slices halfway through the baking time.

In a baking dish, spread a thin layer of marinara sauce.

Arrange a layer of baked eggplant slices on top of the sauce.

Sprinkle shredded mozzarella cheese over the eggplant layer.

Repeat the process, layering marinara sauce, eggplant, and mozzarella until you run out of ingredients, finishing with a layer of cheese on top.

Bake the Eggplant Parmesan in the oven for 25-30 minutes or until the cheese is melted and bubbly, and the edges are golden.

Remove from the oven and let it rest for a few minutes.

Garnish with chopped fresh basil or parsley.

Serve the Eggplant Parmesan hot and enjoy this delicious and gluten-free version of a classic dish!

Quinoa Stuffed Bell Peppers:

Ingredients:

- 4 large bell peppers, halved and seeds removed
- 1 cup quinoa, rinsed
- 2 cups vegetable broth or water
- 1 tablespoon olive oil
- 1 onion, finely chopped
- 2 cloves garlic, minced

- 1 zucchini, diced
- 1 carrot, grated
- 1 cup black beans, drained and rinsed
- 1 cup corn kernels (fresh, frozen, or canned)
- 1 teaspoon ground cumin
- 1 teaspoon chili powder
- Salt and black pepper to taste
- 1 cup tomato sauce
- 1 cup shredded cheese (cheddar, Monterey Jack or a blend)
- Fresh cilantro or parsley for garnish

Instructions:

1. Preheat your oven to 375°F (190°C).
2. In a medium saucepan, combine quinoa and vegetable broth (or water). Bring to a boil then reduce heat to low, cover and simmer for 15-20 minutes or until the quinoa is cooked and water is absorbed.
3. While the quinoa is cooking, heat olive oil in a skillet over medium heat. Add chopped onion and cook until softened.
4. Add minced garlic, diced zucchini and grated carrot to the skillet. Cook for an additional 3-4 minutes until the vegetables are tender.
5. Stir in black beans, corn, ground cumin, chili powder, salt, and black pepper. Cook for another 2-3 minutes to combine the flavors.
6. In a large mixing bowl, combine the cooked quinoa with the vegetable mixture.
7. Spoon the quinoa and vegetable mixture into the halved bell peppers, pressing it down gently.
8. Pour tomato sauce over the stuffed peppers, ensuring they are well covered.
9. Sprinkle shredded cheese over the top of each stuffed pepper.
10. Place the stuffed peppers in a baking dish, cover with foil, and bake in the preheated oven for 25-30 minutes, or until the peppers are tender.

11. Remove the foil and broil for an additional 2-3 minutes until the cheese is melted and bubbly.

12. Garnish with fresh cilantro or parsley.

13. Serve the Quinoa Stuffed Bell Peppers hot, and enjoy this nutritious and flavorful meal!

Vegetarian Chickpea Curry:

Ingredients:

- 2 tablespoons vegetable oil
- 1 large onion, finely chopped
- 3 cloves garlic, minced
- 1 tablespoon fresh ginger, grated
- 1 tablespoon curry powder
- 1 teaspoon ground cumin
- 1 teaspoon ground coriander
- 1 teaspoon turmeric
- 1/2 teaspoon cayenne pepper (adjust to taste)
- 1 can (14 oz) chickpeas, drained and rinsed
- 1 can (14 oz) diced tomatoes
- 1 can (14 oz) coconut milk
- Salt and black pepper to taste
- 2 cups spinach or kale, chopped
- Fresh cilantro, chopped, for garnish
- Cooked rice or naan bread for serving

Instructions:

1. In a large skillet or pot, heat vegetable oil over medium heat.

2. Add chopped onion and cook until softened.

3. Stir in minced garlic and grated ginger, cooking for an additional 1-2 minutes until fragrant.

4. Add curry powder, ground cumin, ground coriander, turmeric, and cayenne pepper to the skillet. Stir well to coat the onions in the spices.

5. Pour in chickpeas, diced tomatoes, and coconut milk. Mix to combine.

6. Season the curry with salt and black pepper to taste. Bring the mixture to a simmer.

7. Reduce the heat to low, cover the skillet, and let it simmer for 15-20 minutes to allow the flavors to meld.

8. Stir in chopped spinach or kale, allowing it to wilt into the curry.

9. Taste and adjust the seasoning if needed.

10. Serve the Vegetarian Chickpea Curry over cooked rice or with naan bread.

Caprese Portobello Mushrooms:

Ingredients:

- 4 large portobello mushrooms, stems removed
- 2 tablespoons balsamic glaze
- 2 tablespoons olive oil
- 4 large tomatoes, sliced
- 8 ounces fresh mozzarella cheese, sliced
- Fresh basil leaves
- Salt and black pepper to taste

Instructions:

1. Preheat your oven to 400°F (200°C).

2. Place the portobello mushrooms on a baking sheet, gill side up.

3. In a small bowl, mix balsamic glaze and olive oil. Brush the mixture over the gill side of each mushroom.

4. Season the mushrooms with salt and black pepper.

5. Bake in the preheated oven for 12-15 minutes or until the mushrooms are tender.

6. While the mushrooms are baking, prepare the toppings. Slice the tomatoes and fresh mozzarella cheese.

7. Once the mushrooms are done, remove them from the oven.

8. On each mushroom, layer slices of tomato and fresh mozzarella.

9. Return the mushrooms to the oven and broil for 2-3 minutes or until the cheese is melted and bubbly.

10. Remove from the oven and garnish with fresh basil leaves.

11. Drizzle additional balsamic glaze over the top if desired.

12. Serve the Caprese Portobello Mushrooms hot, and enjoy.

Mushroom and Spinach Risotto:

Ingredients:

- 1 cup Arborio rice
- 8 cups vegetable or chicken broth, kept warm
- 2 tablespoons olive oil
- 1 onion, finely chopped
- 2 cloves garlic, minced
- 8 oz mushrooms (button or cremini), sliced
- 2 cups fresh spinach, chopped
- 1/2 cup dry white wine
- 1/2 cup grated Parmesan cheese
- Salt and black pepper to taste
- Fresh parsley, chopped, for garnish

Instructions:

1. In a large skillet or wide saucepan, heat olive oil over medium heat.

2. Add chopped onion and cook until softened, about 2-3 minutes.

3. Stir in minced garlic and cook for an additional 1-2 minutes until fragrant.

4. Add sliced mushrooms to the skillet and cook until they release their moisture and become golden brown.

5. Stir in Arborio rice and cook for 1-2 minutes until the rice is lightly toasted.

6. Pour in the dry white wine and stir until most of the liquid is absorbed.

7. Begin adding the warm broth, one ladle at a time, stirring frequently. Allow the liquid to be mostly absorbed before adding the next ladle.

8. Continue this process until the rice is creamy and cooked to al dente texture. This usually takes about 18-20 minutes.

9. In the last few minutes of cooking, stir in chopped fresh spinach until wilted.

10. Once the risotto is done, stir in grated Parmesan cheese. Season with salt and black pepper to taste.

11. Remove the skillet from heat and let it rest for a couple of minutes.

12. Serve the Mushroom and Spinach Risotto hot, garnished with chopped fresh parsley.

Vegetarian Tacos with Avocado Crema:

Ingredients:

For the Avocado Crema:

- 2 ripe avocados, peeled and pitted
- 1/2 cup Greek yogurt or sour cream
- 1 clove garlic, minced
- 1 tablespoon lime juice
- Salt and black pepper to taste

For the Vegetarian Filling:

- 1 tablespoon olive oil
- 1 onion, finely chopped
- 2 bell peppers (any color), thinly sliced
- 1 zucchini, diced
- 1 cup corn kernels (fresh, frozen, or canned)
- 1 can (15 oz) black beans, drained and rinsed
- 1 teaspoon ground cumin
- 1 teaspoon chili powder
- Salt and black pepper to taste

For Assembling:

- Soft taco shells or tortillas
- Shredded lettuce
- Diced tomatoes
- Shredded cheese (cheddar, Monterey Jack, or a blend)
- Fresh cilantro, chopped

Instructions:

1. Prepare the Avocado Crema: In a blender or food processor, combine ripe avocados, Greek yogurt or sour cream, minced garlic, lime juice, salt, and black pepper. Blend until smooth and creamy. Adjust seasoning to taste. Set aside.
2. In a large skillet, heat olive oil over medium heat.
3. Add chopped onion and cook until softened.
4. Stir in thinly sliced bell peppers, diced zucchini, and corn kernels. Cook for 5-7 minutes until the vegetables are tender-crisp.
5. Add drained black beans, ground cumin, chili powder, salt, and black pepper. Stir to combine and cook for an additional 2-3 minutes.
6. Warm the soft taco shells or tortillas according to package instructions.
7. Assemble the tacos by spooning the vegetarian filling onto each shell.
8. Top with shredded lettuce, diced tomatoes, shredded cheese, and fresh cilantro.
9. Drizzle the Avocado Crema over the top.
10. Serve the Vegetarian Tacos with Avocado Crema immediately.

Spinach and Feta Stuffed Mushrooms:

Ingredients:

- 16 large mushrooms, cleaned and stems removed
- 2 cups fresh spinach, chopped
- 1 cup crumbled feta cheese
- 1/4 cup finely chopped red onion
- 2 cloves garlic, minced

- 2 tablespoons olive oil
- Salt and black pepper to taste
- 1/4 cup breadcrumbs (gluten-free if needed)
- Fresh parsley, chopped, for garnish

Instructions:

1. Preheat your oven to 375°F (190°C). Line a baking sheet with parchment paper.
2. Clean the mushrooms and remove the stems. Set aside.
3. In a large skillet, heat olive oil over medium heat.
4. Add minced garlic and chopped red onion to the skillet. Sauté until the onion is softened.
5. Add chopped spinach to the skillet and cook until wilted. Season with salt and black pepper to taste.
6. Remove the skillet from heat and let the spinach mixture cool for a few minutes.
7. In a bowl, combine the spinach mixture with crumbled feta cheese.
8. Place the mushroom caps on the prepared baking sheet.
9. Fill each mushroom cap with the spinach and feta mixture.
10. Sprinkle bread crumbs over the top of each stuffed mushroom.
11. Bake in the preheated oven for 15-20 minutes or until the mushrooms are tender and the tops are golden brown.
12. Garnish with chopped fresh parsley before serving.

Zucchini Noodles with Pesto:

Ingredients:

For the Pesto:

- 2 cups fresh basil leaves, packed
- 1/2 cup grated Parmesan cheese
- 1/3 cup pine nuts or walnuts
- 2 cloves garlic, peeled
- 1/2 cup extra-virgin olive oil

- Salt and black pepper to taste
- Juice of 1 lemon

For the Zucchini Noodles:

- 4 medium-sized zucchini, spiralized into noodles
- 1 tablespoon olive oil
- Cherry tomatoes, halved, for garnish (optional)
- Grated Parmesan cheese, for garnish (optional)

Instructions:

1. Prepare the Pesto: In a food processor, combine basil, grated Parmesan cheese, pine nuts or walnuts, and peeled garlic. Pulse until coarsely chopped.
2. With the food processor running, slowly pour in the olive oil until the pesto reaches your desired consistency.
3. Season the pesto with salt, black pepper, and lemon juice. Pulse once more to combine. Set aside.
4. In a large skillet, heat olive oil over medium heat.
5. Add the spiralized zucchini noodles to the skillet and sauté for 2 3 minutes until they are just tender but still have a slight crunch.
6. Remove the skillet from heat and toss the zucchini noodles with the prepared pesto until evenly coated.
7. Optionally, garnish with halved cherry tomatoes and grated Parmesan cheese.
8. Serve the Zucchini Noodles with Pesto immediately.

Vegetarian Lentil Sloppy Joes:

Ingredients:

- 1 cup dried brown lentils, rinsed and drained
- 3 cups vegetable broth
- 1 tablespoon olive oil
- 1 onion, finely chopped
- 1 bell pepper, finely chopped

- 2 cloves garlic, minced
- 1 can (14 oz) crushed tomatoes
- 1/4 cup tomato paste
- 2 tablespoons soy sauce
- 1 tablespoon Dijon mustard
- 1 tablespoon chili powder
- 1 teaspoon ground cumin
- 1 teaspoon smoked paprika
- 1/2 teaspoon cayenne pepper (adjust to taste)
- Salt and black pepper to taste
- Hamburger buns or rolls for serving

Instructions:

1. In a medium saucepan, combine brown lentils and vegetable broth. Bring to a boil, then reduce heat to low, cover, and simmer for about 25-30 minutes or until lentils are tender but still hold their shape. Drain any excess liquid.
2. In a large skillet, heat olive oil over medium heat.
3. Add chopped onion and bell pepper. Sauté until softened, about 5 minutes.
4. Stir in minced garlic and cook for an additional 1-2 minutes until fragrant.
5. Add cooked lentils to the skillet, along with crushed tomatoes, tomato paste, soy sauce, Dijon mustard, chili powder, ground cumin, smoked paprika, cayenne pepper, salt, and black pepper. Mix well.
6. Simmer the mixture for 10-15 minutes, allowing the flavors to meld and the sauce to thicken.
7. Taste and adjust the seasoning if needed.
8. Serve the Vegetarian Lentil Sloppy Joes on hamburger buns or rolls.

Cauliflower Steak with Chimichurri Sauce:

Ingredients:

For the Cauliflower Steaks:

- 1 large cauliflower head
- 3 tablespoons olive oil
- 1 teaspoon smoked paprika
- 1 teaspoon garlic powder
- Salt and black pepper to taste

For the Chimichurri Sauce:

- 1 cup fresh parsley, finely chopped
- 1/4 cup fresh cilantro, finely chopped
- 3 cloves garlic, minced
- 1/2 teaspoon dried oregano
- 1/2 teaspoon red pepper flakes (adjust to taste)
- 1/4 cup red wine vinegar
- 1/2 cup extra-virgin olive oil
- Salt and black pepper to taste

Instructions:

1. Preheat your oven to 425°F (220°C).
2. Remove the leaves from the cauliflower head, and trim the stem end, leaving the core intact.
3. Slice the cauliflower into 1-inch thick steaks. You can get about 2-3 steaks from one cauliflower head, depending on its size.
4. In a small bowl, mix olive oil, smoked paprika, garlic powder, salt, and black pepper to create a marinade.
5. Brush both sides of each cauliflower steak with the marinade.
6. Place the cauliflower steaks on a baking sheet lined with parchment paper.
7. Roast in the preheated oven for 25-30 minutes, flipping the steaks halfway through, or until the cauliflower is golden and tender.
8. While the cauliflower is roasting, prepare the Chimichurri Sauce. In a bowl, combine finely chopped parsley, finely chopped cilantro, minced garlic, dried

oregano, red pepper flakes, red wine vinegar, and extra-virgin olive oil. Mix well. Season with salt and black pepper to taste.

9. Once the cauliflower steaks are done, transfer them to serving plates.

10. Spoon the Chimichurri Sauce over the cauliflower steaks or serve it on the side.

Vegetarian Thai Green Curry:

Ingredients:

- 2 tablespoons green curry paste
- 1 can (14 oz) coconut milk
- 1 cup vegetable broth
- 1 tablespoon soy sauce
- 1 tablespoon brown sugar
- 1 tablespoon vegetable oil
- 1 onion, thinly sliced
- 1 bell pepper, thinly sliced
- 1 zucchini, sliced into half-moons
- 1 carrot, julienned
- 1 cup broccoli florets
- 1 cup firm tofu, cubed
- Fresh basil leaves, for garnish
- Cooked jasmine rice, for serving

Instructions:

1. In a large pot or wok, heat vegetable oil over medium heat.

2. Add green curry paste to the pot and stir-fry for 1-2 minutes until fragrant.

3. Pour in coconut milk, vegetable broth, soy sauce, and brown sugar. Stir well to combine.

4. Bring the mixture to a simmer, then reduce the heat to low.

5. Add sliced onion, bell pepper, zucchini, julienned carrot, broccoli florets, and cubed tofu to the pot. Simmer for 10-15 minutes or until the vegetables are tender.

6. Taste and adjust the seasoning if needed, adding more soy sauce or brown sugar according to your preference.

7. Remove the pot from heat.

8. Serve the Vegetarian Thai Green Curry over cooked jasmine rice.

Vegan Ideas:

Vegan Chickpea Salad Wraps:

Ingredients:

For the Chickpea Salad:

- 2 cans (15 oz each) chickpeas, drained and rinsed
- 1/4 cup vegan mayonnaise
- 1 tablespoon Dijon mustard
- 2 tablespoons lemon juice
- 1 celery stalk, finely chopped
- 1/4 cup red onion, finely chopped
- 1/4 cup fresh parsley, chopped
- Salt and black pepper to taste

For the Wraps:

- Whole-grain or gluten-free wraps
- Lettuce leaves
- Sliced tomatoes
- Sliced cucumbers
- Avocado slices (optional)
- Alfalfa sprouts or microgreens (optional)

Instructions:

1. In a large bowl, mash the chickpeas with a fork or potato masher. Leave some chunks for texture.

2. Add vegan mayonnaise, Dijon mustard, lemon juice, chopped celery, chopped red onion, and chopped fresh parsley to the mashed chickpeas. Mix well to combine.

3. Season the chickpea salad with salt and black pepper to taste. Adjust the seasoning if needed.

4. Lay out a wrap and place a lettuce leaf in the center.

5. Spoon a generous amount of the chickpea salad onto the lettuce.

6. Add sliced tomatoes, sliced cucumbers, avocado slices (if using), and alfalfa sprouts or microgreens.

7. Fold the sides of the wrap over the filling, then roll it up tightly.

8. Repeat with the remaining wraps.

9. Slice the wraps in half if desired.

10. Serve the Vegan Chickpea Salad Wraps immediately.

Vegan Buddha Bowl:

Ingredients:

For the Quinoa:

- 1 cup quinoa, rinsed
- 2 cups vegetable broth
- Salt to taste

For the Roasted Vegetables:

- 1 sweet potato, peeled and diced
- 1 cup broccoli florets
- 1 cup cherry tomatoes, halved
- 1 tablespoon olive oil
- Salt and black pepper to taste
- 1 teaspoon smoked paprika
- 1/2 teaspoon garlic powder

For the Lemon-Tahini Dressing:

- 1/4 cup tahini

- 2 tablespoons olive oil

- 2 tablespoons lemon juice

- 1 tablespoon maple syrup

- 1 clove garlic, minced

- Salt and black pepper to taste

- Water (as needed to thin)

For Assembly:

- 1 avocado, sliced

- 1 cup canned chickpeas, drained and rinsed

- Mixed greens or spinach

- Sesame seeds for garnish (optional)

- Fresh herbs, chopped (cilantro, parsley, or mint)

Instructions:

1. Preheat your oven to 425°F (220°C).

2. Rinse quinoa under cold water. In a saucepan, combine quinoa, vegetable broth, and a pinch of salt. Bring to a boil, then reduce heat to low, cover, and simmer for 15-20 minutes or until quinoa is cooked and water is absorbed.

3. Toss diced sweet potato, broccoli florets, and cherry tomatoes with olive oil, salt, black pepper, smoked paprika, and garlic powder.

4. Spread the vegetables on a baking sheet in a single layer. Roast in the preheated oven for 20-25 minutes or until the vegetables are tender and golden.

5. In a small bowl, whisk together tahini, olive oil, lemon juice, maple syrup, minced garlic, salt, and black pepper. Add water as needed to achieve the desired dressing consistency.

6. Assemble the Buddha Bowl: Divide cooked quinoa among serving bowls. Arrange roasted vegetables, avocado slices, chickpeas, and mixed greens on top.

7. Drizzle the Lemon-Tahini Dressing over the bowl.

8. Garnish with sesame seeds and fresh herbs.

9. Serve the Vegan Buddha Bowl immediately and enjoy.

Vegan Lentil Soup:

Ingredients:

- 1 cup dried green or brown lentils, rinsed and drained
- 1 tablespoon olive oil
- 1 onion, finely chopped
- 2 carrots, diced
- 2 celery stalks, diced
- 3 cloves garlic, minced
- 1 teaspoon ground cumin
- 1 teaspoon ground coriander
- 1 teaspoon smoked paprika
- 1/2 teaspoon ground turmeric
- 1/4 teaspoon cayenne pepper (optional, for heat)
- 1 can (14 oz) diced tomatoes
- 6 cups vegetable broth
- 1 bay leaf
- Salt and black pepper to taste
- Juice of 1 lemon
- Fresh parsley, chopped, for garnish

Instructions:

1. In a large pot, heat olive oil over medium heat.
2. Add chopped onion, diced carrots, and diced celery. Sauté until the vegetables are softened, about 5-7 minutes.
3. Stir in minced garlic and cook for an additional 1-2 minutes until fragrant.
4. Add ground cumin, ground coriander, smoked paprika, ground turmeric, and cayenne pepper (if using). Mix well to coat the vegetables in the spices.
5. Pour in diced tomatoes and vegetable broth. Add rinsed lentils and bay leaf. Stir to combine.

6. Bring the soup to a boil, then reduce the heat to low, cover, and simmer for 25-30 minutes or until the lentils are tender.

7. Season the soup with salt and black pepper to taste.

8. Stir in lemon juice just before serving to brighten the flavors.

9. Remove the bay leaf.

10. Ladle the Vegan Lentil Soup into bowls and garnish with chopped fresh parsley.

11. Serve hot and enjoy this hearty and nutritious plant-based soup!

Stuffed Acorn Squash:

Ingredients:

- 2 acorn squash, halved and seeds removed
- 1 tablespoon olive oil
- Salt and black pepper to taste

For the Filling:

- 1 cup quinoa, rinsed
- 2 cups vegetable broth
- 1 tablespoon olive oil
- 1 onion, finely chopped
- 2 cloves garlic, minced
- 1 apple, diced
- 1/2 cup dried cranberries or raisins
- 1/2 cup chopped pecans or walnuts
- 1 teaspoon dried sage
- 1 teaspoon dried thyme
- Salt and black pepper to taste

Instructions:

1. Preheat your oven to 400°F (200°C).

2. Rub the cut sides of the acorn squash with olive oil. Season with salt and black pepper.

3. Place the squash halves cut side down on a baking sheet.

4. Roast in the preheated oven for 30-40 minutes or until the squash is tender when pierced with a fork.

5. While the squash is roasting, prepare the quinoa. In a saucepan, combine quinoa and vegetable broth. Bring to a boil, then reduce heat to low, cover, and simmer for 15-20 minutes or until quinoa is cooked and liquid is absorbed.

6. In a skillet, heat olive oil over medium heat. Add chopped onion and cook until softened.

7. Stir in minced garlic, diced apple, dried cranberries or raisins, chopped nuts, dried sage, dried thyme, salt, and black pepper. Cook for an additional 3-4 minutes until the apples are tender.

8. Mix the cooked quinoa with the apple and nut mixture, combining well.

9. Once the acorn squash halves are done roasting, fill each half with the quinoa mixture.

10. Return the filled squash halves to the oven and bake for an additional 10-15 minutes.

11. Serve the Stuffed Acorn Squash hot.

Vegan Pad Thai:

Ingredients:

For the Pad Thai Sauce:

- 1/4 cup soy sauce or tamari (for gluten-free)
- 2 tablespoons maple syrup or agave nectar
- 1 tablespoon rice vinegar
- 1 tablespoon tamarind paste
- 1 teaspoon sriracha or chili sauce (adjust to taste)

For the Pad Thai:

- 8 oz rice noodles, soaked according to package instructions
- 2 tablespoons vegetable oil

- 1 block (about 14 oz) firm tofu, pressed and cubed
- 1 cup broccoli florets
- 1 carrot, julienned
- 1 red bell pepper, thinly sliced
- 2 cloves garlic, minced
- 1 cup bean sprouts
- 3 green onions, sliced
- 1/4 cup chopped peanuts
- Lime wedges for serving
- Fresh cilantro for garnish (optional)

Instructions:

1. In a small bowl, whisk together soy sauce or tamari, maple syrup or agave nectar, rice vinegar, tamarind paste, and sriracha. Set aside.
2. Cook rice noodles according to package instructions. Drain and set aside.
3. In a large wok or skillet, heat vegetable oil over medium-high heat.
4. Add cubed tofu and cook until golden brown on all sides. Remove tofu from the pan and set aside.
5. In the same pan, add more oil if needed. Sauté broccoli, julienned carrot, and sliced red bell pepper until vegetables are tender-crisp.
6. Push the vegetables to one side of the pan and add minced garlic to the other side. Sauté for 30 seconds until fragrant.
7. Add cooked rice noodles, tofu, and prepared Pad Thai sauce to the pan. Toss everything together until well coated and heated through.
8. Stir in bean sprouts and sliced green onions. Cook for an additional 1-2 minutes.
9. Remove from heat and garnish with chopped peanuts.
10. Serve Vegan Pad Thai hot, garnished with lime wedges and fresh cilantro if desired.

Vegan Cauliflower Buffalo Wings:

Ingredients:

For the Cauliflower Wings:

- 1 large head of cauliflower, cut into florets
- 1 cup all-purpose flour (or chickpea flour for a gluten-free option)
- 1 cup plant-based milk (such as almond, soy, or oat)
- 1 teaspoon garlic powder
- 1 teaspoon onion powder
- 1/2 teaspoon smoked paprika
- Salt and black pepper to taste

For the Buffalo Sauce:

- 1/2 cup hot sauce (such as Frank's RedHot)
- 1/4 cup vegan butter
- 1 tablespoon apple cider vinegar
- 1/2 teaspoon garlic powder
- 1/2 teaspoon onion powder
- 1/2 teaspoon smoked paprika

Instructions:

1. Preheat your oven to 450°F (230°C). Line a baking sheet with parchment paper.
2. In a large bowl, whisk together flour, plant-based milk, garlic powder, onion powder, smoked paprika, salt, and black pepper to create a batter.
3. Dip each cauliflower floret into the batter, ensuring it's well coated, and place it on the prepared baking sheet. Repeat for all florets.
4. Bake in the preheated oven for 20-25 minutes or until the cauliflower is golden brown and crispy.
5. While the cauliflower is baking, prepare the Buffalo sauce. In a small saucepan over low heat, melt vegan butter. Stir in hot sauce, apple cider vinegar, garlic powder, onion powder, and smoked paprika. Simmer for a few minutes until well combined.

6. Once the cauliflower is done baking, transfer the florets to a large bowl.

7. Pour the Buffalo sauce over the cauliflower and toss until the florets are evenly coated.

8. Return the coated cauliflower to the baking sheet and bake for an additional 10-15 minutes or until the sauce is sticky and caramelized.

9. Remove from the oven and let the cauliflower cool for a few minutes.

Vegan Eggplant Lasagna:

Ingredients:

For the Eggplant Slices:

- 2 large eggplants, thinly sliced lengthwise
- Olive oil for brushing
- Salt and black pepper to taste

For the Vegan Ricotta Filling:

- 2 cups raw cashews, soaked in hot water for 1-2 hours
- 1/2 cup nutritional yeast
- 3 tablespoons lemon juice
- 2 cloves garlic, minced
- 1 teaspoon dried basil
- 1 teaspoon dried oregano
- Salt and black pepper to taste

For the Tomato Sauce:

- **2 tablespoons olive oil**
- 1 onion, finely chopped
- 3 cloves garlic, minced
- 1 can (28 oz) crushed tomatoes
- 1 teaspoon dried oregano
- 1 teaspoon dried basil
- Salt and black pepper to taste

For Assembly:

- Vegan mozzarella cheese, shredded
- Fresh basil leaves for garnish (optional)

Instructions:

1. Preheat your oven to 375°F (190°C).
2. Brush the sliced eggplants with olive oil on both sides. Season with salt and black pepper.
3. Arrange the eggplant slices in a single layer on baking sheets. Bake in the preheated oven for 15-20 minutes or until the slices are softened and slightly golden. Set aside.
4. In a food processor, combine soaked cashews, nutritional yeast, lemon juice, minced garlic, dried basil, dried oregano, salt, and black pepper. Blend until you achieve a smooth and creamy consistency. Set aside.
5. In a large skillet, heat olive oil over medium heat. Add chopped onion and cook until softened.
6. Stir in minced garlic and cook for an additional 1-2 minutes until fragrant.
7. Add crushed tomatoes, dried oregano, dried basil, salt, and black pepper to the skillet. Simmer for about 15-20 minutes, allowing the flavors to meld.
8. To assemble the lasagna, spread a thin layer of tomato sauce on the bottom of a baking dish.
9. Place a layer of roasted eggplant slices on top of the sauce.
10. Spread a layer of the vegan ricotta filling over the eggplant slices.
11. Repeat the layers, finishing with a layer of tomato sauce on top.
12. Sprinkle shredded vegan mozzarella cheese over the lasagna.
13. Bake in the preheated oven for 25-30 minutes or until the lasagna is bubbly and the cheese is melted and golden.
14. Remove from the oven and let it cool for a few minutes before serving.
15. Garnish with fresh basil leaves if desired.

Vegan Sweet Potato and Black Bean Quesadillas:

Ingredients:

- 2 large sweet potatoes, peeled and diced
- 1 can (15 oz) black beans, drained and rinsed
- 1 cup corn kernels (fresh, frozen, or canned)
- 1 red bell pepper, diced
- 1 teaspoon ground cumin
- 1 teaspoon chili powder
- Salt and black pepper to taste
- 4 large whole-grain or gluten-free tortillas
- 1 1/2 cups shredded vegan cheese (cheddar or a Mexican blend)
- Fresh cilantro, chopped, for garnish
- Avocado slices for serving (optional)
- Salsa for serving (optional)

Instructions:

1. Steam or boil the diced sweet potatoes until they are fork-tender. Drain and set aside.
2. In a large bowl, combine the steamed sweet potatoes, black beans, corn, diced red bell pepper, ground cumin, chili powder, salt, and black pepper. Mix well.
3. Preheat a large skillet or griddle over medium heat.
4. Place a tortilla on the hot skillet. Spread a portion of the sweet potato and black bean mixture evenly over half of the tortilla.
5. Sprinkle a generous amount of shredded vegan cheese over the filling.
6. Fold the other half of the tortilla over the filling, creating a half-moon shape.
7. Cook the quesadilla for 2-3 minutes on each side or until the tortilla is golden brown and the cheese is melted.
8. Repeat the process with the remaining tortillas and filling.
9. Once all quesadillas are cooked, transfer them to a cutting board and let them rest for a minute before slicing.

10. Garnish with chopped fresh cilantro.

11. Serve the Sweet Potato and Black Bean Quesadillas with avocado slices and salsa.

Vegan Spinach and Artichoke Stuffed Peppers:

Ingredients:

- 4 large bell peppers, halved and seeds removed
- 1 tablespoon olive oil
- 1 onion, finely chopped
- 3 cloves garlic, minced
- 2 cups fresh spinach, chopped
- 1 can (14 oz) artichoke hearts, drained and chopped
- 1 cup raw cashews, soaked in hot water for 1-2 hours
- 1/2 cup nutritional yeast
- 1 tablespoon lemon juice
- Salt and black pepper to taste
- 1 cup cooked quinoa or rice
- Vegan mozzarella cheese, shredded, for topping (optional)
- Fresh parsley, chopped, for garnish

Instructions:

1. Preheat your oven to 375°F (190°C).

2. Heat olive oil in a large skillet over medium heat. Add chopped onion and sauté until softened.

3. Stir in minced garlic and cook for an additional 1-2 minutes until fragrant.

4. Add chopped fresh spinach to the skillet and cook until wilted.

5. In a food processor, combine soaked cashews, nutritional yeast, lemon juice, salt, and black pepper. Blend until you achieve a smooth and creamy consistency.

6. Transfer the cashew mixture to the skillet with the sautéed vegetables. Add chopped artichoke hearts and cooked quinoa or rice. Mix well to combine.

7. Taste and adjust the seasoning if needed.

8. Arrange the halved bell peppers in a baking dish.

9. Stuff each pepper half with the spinach and artichoke mixture.

10. If desired, sprinkle vegan mozzarella cheese on top of each stuffed pepper.

11. Cover the baking dish with aluminum foil and bake in the preheated oven for 25-30 minutes or until the peppers are tender.

12. Remove the foil and bake for an additional 5-10 minutes until the cheese (if used) is melted and bubbly.

13. Garnish with chopped fresh parsley.

Vegan Tofu Stir-Fry:

Ingredients:

For the Tofu Marinade:
- 1 block (about 14 oz) extra-firm tofu, pressed and cubed
- 3 tablespoons soy sauce or tamari
- 1 tablespoon maple syrup or agave nectar
- 1 tablespoon rice vinegar
- 1 teaspoon sesame oil
- 1 teaspoon cornstarch

For the Stir-Fry Sauce:
- 1/4 cup soy sauce or tamari
- 2 tablespoons hoisin sauce
- 1 tablespoon maple syrup or agave nectar
- 1 tablespoon rice vinegar
- 1 teaspoon sesame oil

For the Stir-Fry:
- 2 tablespoons vegetable oil
- 1 onion, thinly sliced
- 2 bell peppers, thinly sliced
- 1 carrot, julienned
- 2 cups broccoli florets
- 2 cups snap peas, ends trimmed
- 3 cloves garlic, minced
- 1 tablespoon ginger, grated
- Cooked brown rice or noodles for serving

- Sesame seeds and green onions for garnish

Instructions:

1. In a bowl, whisk together the tofu marinade ingredients: soy sauce, maple syrup, rice vinegar, sesame oil, and cornstarch.
2. Add the cubed tofu to the marinade, ensuring each piece is well coated. Let it marinate for at least 30 minutes.
3. In another bowl, mix together the stir-fry sauce ingredients: soy sauce, hoisin sauce, maple syrup, rice vinegar, and sesame oil. Set aside.
4. Heat vegetable oil in a wok or large skillet over medium-high heat.
5. Add marinated tofu cubes to the hot pan, reserving the marinade. Cook until the tofu is golden and slightly crispy on all sides. Remove tofu from the pan and set aside.
6. In the same pan, add a bit more oil if needed. Sauté sliced onion, bell peppers, julienned carrot, broccoli florets, and snap peas until they are tender-crisp.
7. Add minced garlic and grated ginger to the vegetables, stirring for about 1-2 minutes until fragrant.
8. Pour the reserved tofu marinade over the vegetables and stir to combine.
9. Return the cooked tofu to the pan and pour the prepared stir-fry sauce over everything. Stir well to coat everything evenly.
10. Cook for an additional 2-3 minutes until the sauce thickens slightly.
11. Serve the Vegan Tofu Stir-Fry over cooked brown rice or noodles.

Vegan Jackfruit Tacos:

Ingredients:

For the Jackfruit Filling:

- 2 cans (20 oz each) young green jackfruit in water or brine, drained and rinsed
- 2 tablespoons olive oil
- 1 onion, finely chopped
- 3 cloves garlic, minced
- 1 teaspoon ground cumin
- 1 teaspoon smoked paprika
- 1/2 teaspoon chili powder
- 1/2 teaspoon onion powder
- 1/2 teaspoon garlic powder
- Salt and black pepper to taste
- 1/2 cup vegetable broth

- 1/4 cup tomato paste
- 1 tablespoon soy sauce or tamari
- 1 tablespoon maple syrup or agave nectar

For Serving:

- Corn or flour tortillas
- Shredded lettuce
- Diced tomatoes
- Sliced avocado
- Fresh cilantro, chopped
- Lime wedges

Instructions:

1. Rinse and drain the canned jackfruit. Using your fingers or a fork, shred the jackfruit into pieces that resemble shredded meat.
2. In a large skillet, heat olive oil over medium heat. Add chopped onion and cook until softened.
3. Stir in minced garlic and cook for an additional 1-2 minutes until fragrant.
4. Add the shredded jackfruit to the skillet, along with ground cumin, smoked paprika, chili powder, onion powder, garlic powder, salt, and black pepper. Toss to coat the jackfruit in the spices.
5. Pour vegetable broth, tomato paste, soy sauce or tamari, and maple syrup or agave nectar over the jackfruit. Stir well to combine.
6. Simmer the jackfruit mixture over medium-low heat for 15-20 minutes, stirring occasionally. The jackfruit should absorb the flavors and soften.
7. Adjust the seasoning if needed and cook for an additional 5-10 minutes until the jackfruit has a meat-like texture.
8. Warm the tortillas according to package instructions.
9. Assemble the Vegan Jackfruit Tacos by spooning the jackfruit filling onto the tortillas.
10. Top with shredded lettuce, diced tomatoes, sliced avocado, and chopped fresh cilantro.
11. Serve the tacos with lime wedges for squeezing over the top.
12. Enjoy these flavorful and plant-based Jackfruit Tacos as a delicious meatless alternative!

CHAPTER 7: SIDES AND SNACKS

Roasted Garlic Mashed Potatoes:

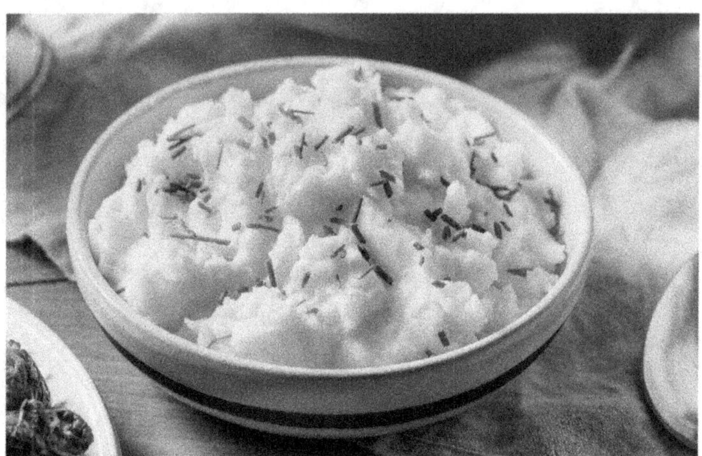

Ingredients:

- **4 lbs (about 1**.8 kg) potatoes, peeled and cut into chunks
- 1 whole head of garlic
- Olive oil for roasting
- 1 cup unsweetened almond milk (or any plant-based milk)
- 1/2 cup vegan butter
- Salt and black pepper to taste
- Chopped fresh chives or parsley for garnish (optional)

Instructions:

1. Preheat your oven to 400°F (200°C).
2. Cut the top off the head of garlic, exposing the cloves. Place the garlic on a piece of foil, drizzle with olive oil, and wrap it tightly.

3. Roast the wrapped garlic in the preheated oven for about 30-40 minutes or until the cloves are soft and golden brown. Remove from the oven and let it cool.

4. While the garlic is roasting, peel and cut the potatoes into chunks.

5. Boil the potato chunks in a large pot of salted water until they are fork-tender, about 15-20 minutes.

6. Drain the potatoes and return them to the pot.

7. Squeeze the roasted garlic cloves out of their skins and add them to the pot with the potatoes.

8. Add vegan butter and almond milk to the pot.

9. Mash the potatoes and roasted garlic until smooth and creamy. You can use a potato masher or a hand mixer for a smoother consistency.

10. Season the mashed potatoes with salt and black pepper to taste. Adjust the consistency with more almond milk if needed.

11. Continue mashing until you reach your desired smoothness.

12. Transfer the Roasted Garlic Mashed Potatoes to a serving dish.

13. Garnish with chopped fresh chives or parsley if desired.

Gluten-Free Garlic Bread:

Ingredients:

- 1 loaf gluten-free bread (store-bought or homemade)
- 1/2 cup (1 stick) vegan butter, softened
- 4 cloves garlic, minced
- 2 tablespoons fresh parsley, finely chopped
- Salt to taste

Instructions:

1. Preheat your oven according to the instructions on the gluten-free bread package or recipe.

2. Slice the gluten-free bread into your desired thickness.

3. In a small bowl, combine softened vegan butter, minced garlic, chopped fresh parsley, and a pinch of salt. Mix well to create the garlic butter spread.

4. Spread the garlic butter mixture evenly over each slice of gluten-free bread.

5. Place the garlic buttered slices on a baking sheet or in an oven-safe dish.

6. Bake in the preheated oven according to the instructions on the gluten-free bread package or recipe, or until the edges are golden brown.

7. Keep an eye on the bread while it's baking, as gluten-free bread may have different baking times.

8. Once the gluten-free garlic bread is baked to perfection, remove it from the oven.

9. Serve the Gluten-Free Garlic Bread warm.

Sauteed Lemon Asparagus:

Ingredients:

- 1 bunch fresh asparagus, tough ends trimmed
- 2 tablespoons olive oil
- 2 cloves garlic, minced
- Zest of 1 lemon
- Juice of 1 lemon
- Salt and black pepper to taste
- Optional: Grated Parmesan cheese for garnish

Instructions:

1. Heat olive oil in a large skillet over medium heat.

2. Add minced garlic to the skillet and sauté for about 1 minute until fragrant.

3. Add the trimmed asparagus spears to the skillet. Cook for 3-5 minutes, stirring occasionally, until the asparagus is crisp-tender.

4. Zest the lemon directly into the skillet, and then squeeze the lemon juice over the asparagus.

5. Continue to sauté the asparagus for an additional 2-3 minutes, allowing the flavors to meld.

6. Season the sautéed asparagus with salt and black pepper to taste. Adjust the seasoning if needed.

7. Optional: Garnish with grated Parmesan cheese for added flavor.

8. Transfer the Sauteed Lemon Asparagus to a serving platter.

Quinoa Pilaf with Vegetables:

Ingredients:

- 1 cup quinoa, rinsed
- 2 cups vegetable broth
- 1 tablespoon olive oil
- 1 onion, finely chopped
- 2 cloves garlic, minced
- 1 carrot, diced
- 1 zucchini, diced
- 1 red bell pepper, diced
- 1 cup frozen peas
- 1 teaspoon ground cumin
- 1 teaspoon ground coriander
- Salt and black pepper to taste
- Fresh parsley or cilantro, chopped, for garnish

Instructions:

1. Rinse the quinoa under cold water.

2. In a saucepan, combine quinoa and vegetable broth. Bring to a boil, then reduce heat to low, cover, and simmer for 15-20 minutes or until quinoa is cooked and liquid is absorbed.

3. While the quinoa is cooking, heat olive oil in a large skillet over medium heat.

4. Add chopped onion and sauté until softened.

5. Stir in minced garlic and cook for an additional 1-2 minutes until fragrant.

6. Add diced carrot, zucchini, red bell pepper, and frozen peas to the skillet. Cook for 5-7 minutes or until the vegetables are tender-crisp.

7. Sprinkle ground cumin and ground coriander over the vegetables. Season with salt and black pepper to taste. Stir well to combine.

8. Once the quinoa is done cooking, fluff it with a fork and add it to the skillet with the sautéed vegetables. Mix everything together.

9. Adjust the seasoning if needed.

10. Garnish the Quinoa Pilaf with chopped fresh parsley or cilantro.

Cauliflower Rice with Herbs:

Ingredients:

- 1 head cauliflower, washed and dried
- 2 tablespoons olive oil
- 2 cloves garlic, minced
- 1 teaspoon dried thyme
- 1 teaspoon dried rosemary
- Salt and black pepper to taste
- Fresh parsley, chopped, for garnish

Instructions:

1. Cut the cauliflower into florets, removing the tough stem.

2. In batches, pulse the cauliflower florets in a food processor until they resemble the texture of rice. Be careful not to overprocess; you want a rice-like consistency.

3. Heat olive oil in a large skillet over medium heat.

4. Add minced garlic to the skillet and sauté for about 1 minute until fragrant.

5. Add the cauliflower rice to the skillet, spreading it evenly.

6. Sprinkle dried thyme and dried rosemary over the cauliflower rice. Season with salt and black pepper to taste.

7. Stir well to combine and sauté the cauliflower rice for 5-7 minutes, stirring occasionally. The goal is to cook it until it's tender but not mushy.

8. Adjust the seasoning if needed.

9. Garnish the Cauliflower Rice with chopped fresh parsley.

Gluten-Free Cornbread:

Ingredients:

- 1 cup gluten-free cornmeal
- 1 cup gluten-free all-purpose flour
- 1 tablespoon baking powder
- 1/2 teaspoon baking soda
- 1/2 teaspoon salt
- 1 cup non-dairy milk (such as almond or soy milk)
- 1/4 cup maple syrup or agave nectar
- 1/4 cup vegetable oil
- 2 flax eggs (2 tablespoons ground flaxseed mixed with 6 tablespoons water)
- Optional: 1/2 cup corn kernels (fresh, frozen, or canned)

Instructions:

1. Preheat your oven to 400°F (200°C). Grease a square or round baking pan.

2. In a small bowl, prepare the flax eggs by mixing ground flaxseed with water. Set aside to thicken.

3. In a large mixing bowl, whisk together gluten-free cornmeal, gluten-free all-purpose flour, baking powder, baking soda, and salt.

4. In another bowl, combine non-dairy milk, maple syrup or agave nectar, vegetable oil, and the prepared flax eggs.

5. Pour the wet ingredients into the dry ingredients and stir until just combined. Avoid overmixing.

6. If desired, fold in corn kernels into the batter.

7. Pour the batter into the prepared baking pan, spreading it evenly.

8. Bake in the preheated oven for 20-25 minutes or until a toothpick inserted into the center comes out clean.

9. Remove from the oven and let the gluten-free cornbread cool in the pan for a few minutes before transferring it to a wire rack to cool completely.

10. Once cooled, slice and serve the Gluten-Free Cornbread.

Balsamic Glazed Brussels Sprouts:

Ingredients:

- 1 lb Brussels sprouts, trimmed and halved
- 2 tablespoons olive oil
- Salt and black pepper to taste
- 2 tablespoons balsamic vinegar
- 1 tablespoon maple syrup or agave nectar
- 1/4 cup chopped pecans or walnuts (optional)
- Fresh parsley, chopped, for garnish (optional)

Instructions:

1. Preheat your oven to 400°F (200°C).

2. In a large bowl, toss the trimmed and halved Brussels sprouts with olive oil, salt, and black pepper until evenly coated.

3. Spread the Brussels sprouts in a single layer on a baking sheet.

4. Roast in the preheated oven for 20-25 minutes or until the Brussels sprouts are golden brown and crispy on the edges. Shake the pan or stir the Brussels sprouts halfway through the cooking time for even roasting.

5. While the Brussels sprouts are roasting, prepare the balsamic glaze. In a small saucepan, combine balsamic vinegar and maple syrup or agave nectar. Bring to a simmer over medium heat and cook for 3-5 minutes until the mixture has reduced and thickened slightly.

6. Once the Brussels sprouts are done roasting, transfer them to a bowl.

7. Drizzle the balsamic glaze over the roasted Brussels sprouts and toss to coat evenly.

8. If using, sprinkle chopped pecans or walnuts over the Brussels sprouts and toss again.

9. Garnish with fresh chopped parsley if desired.

Vegan Coleslaw:

Ingredients:

For the Coleslaw:

- 1 small green cabbage, finely shredded
- 2 large carrots, grated
- 1 red onion, thinly sliced

For the Vegan Coleslaw Dressing:

- 1 cup vegan mayonnaise
- 2 tablespoons Dijon mustard
- 2 tablespoons apple cider vinegar
- 2 tablespoons maple syrup or agave nectar
- Salt and black pepper to taste

Optional Add-ins:

- 1/2 cup raisins or dried cranberries
- 1/4 cup chopped fresh parsley or cilantro

Instructions:

1. In a large mixing bowl, combine shredded green cabbage, grated carrots, and thinly sliced red onion.

2. In a separate bowl, whisk together vegan mayonnaise, Dijon mustard, apple cider vinegar, maple syrup or agave nectar, salt, and black pepper. Adjust the seasoning to your taste.

3. Pour the dressing over the shredded vegetables.

4. Toss the coleslaw until the dressing evenly coats the vegetables.

5. If desired, add optional add-ins such as raisins or dried cranberries for sweetness and chopped fresh parsley or cilantro for freshness.

6. Cover the Vegan Coleslaw and refrigerate for at least 30 minutes to allow the flavors to meld.

7. Before serving, give the coleslaw a final toss to ensure it's well coated in the dressing.

Gluten-Free Stuffing:

Ingredients:

- 1 loaf gluten-free bread, cubed and dried (leave out overnight or toast in the oven)
- 1/2 cup (1 stick) vegan butter
- 1 large onion, finely chopped
- 3 celery stalks, finely chopped
- 3 cloves garlic, minced
- 1 teaspoon dried thyme
- 1 teaspoon dried sage
- 1 teaspoon dried rosemary
- 1 teaspoon dried parsley
- Salt and black pepper to taste
- 2 to 2 1/2 cups gluten-free vegetable broth
- 2 flax eggs (2 tablespoons ground flaxseed mixed with 6 tablespoons water)
- Chopped fresh parsley for garnish (optional)

Instructions:

1. Preheat your oven to 350°F (175°C). Grease a baking dish.
2. In a large skillet, melt vegan butter over medium heat.
3. Add chopped onion and celery to the skillet. Sauté until the vegetables are softened, about 5-7 minutes.
4. Stir in minced garlic and cook for an additional 1-2 minutes until fragrant.
5. Add dried thyme, sage, rosemary, parsley, salt, and black pepper to the skillet. Mix well to combine.

6. In a large mixing bowl, combine the dried gluten-free bread cubes and the sautéed vegetable mixture.

7. In a separate bowl, prepare the flax eggs by mixing ground flaxseed with water. Let it sit for a few minutes until it thickens.

8. Pour the flax eggs over the bread and vegetables, tossing everything to coat evenly.

9. Gradually pour gluten-free vegetable broth over the mixture, stirring as you go. Add enough broth to moisten the stuffing to your desired consistency.

10. Transfer the gluten-free stuffing to the greased baking dish, spreading it evenly.

11. Cover the baking dish with aluminum foil and bake in the preheated oven for 30 minutes.

12. Remove the foil and bake for an additional 15-20 minutes or until the top is golden brown and crispy.

13. Garnish with chopped fresh parsley if desired.

Roasted Sweet Potato Wedges:

Ingredients:

- **3 large sweet potatoes**, peeled and cut into wedges
- 2 tablespoons olive oil
- 1 teaspoon smoked paprika
- 1 teaspoon garlic powder
- 1 teaspoon onion powder
- 1/2 teaspoon ground cumin
- 1/2 teaspoon chili powder
- Salt and black pepper to taste
- Fresh parsley, chopped, for garnish (optional)

Instructions:

1. Preheat your oven to 425°F (220°C).

2. In a large bowl, toss the sweet potato wedges with olive oil until evenly coated.

3. In a small bowl, mix smoked paprika, garlic powder, onion powder, ground cumin, chili powder, salt, and black pepper.

4. Sprinkle the spice mixture over the sweet potato wedges, tossing to ensure they are well-seasoned.

5. Arrange the seasoned sweet potato wedges in a single layer on a baking sheet.

6. Roast in the preheated oven for 25-30 minutes, flipping the wedges halfway through, or until the edges are crispy and golden brown.

7. Remove from the oven and let them cool slightly.

8. Garnish with chopped fresh parsley if desired.

Caprese Quinoa Salad:

Ingredients:

- 1 loaf gluten-free bread, cubed and dried (leave out overnight or toast in the oven)
- 1/2 cup (1 stick) vegan butter
- 1 large onion, finely chopped
- 3 celery stalks, finely chopped
- 3 cloves garlic, minced
- 1 teaspoon dried thyme
- 1 teaspoon dried sage
- 1 teaspoon dried rosemary
- 1 teaspoon dried parsley
- Salt and black pepper to taste
- 2 to 2 1/2 cups gluten-free vegetable broth
- 2 flax eggs (2 tablespoons ground flaxseed mixed with 6 tablespoons water)
- Chopped fresh parsley for garnish (optional)

Instructions:

1. Preheat your oven to 350°F (175°C). Grease a baking dish.

2. In a large skillet, melt vegan butter over medium heat.

3. Add chopped onion and celery to the skillet. Sauté until the vegetables are softened, about 5-7 minutes.

4. Stir in minced garlic and cook for an additional 1-2 minutes until fragrant.

5. Add dried thyme, sage, rosemary, parsley, salt, and black pepper to the skillet. Mix well to combine.

6. In a large mixing bowl, combine the dried gluten-free bread cubes and the sautéed vegetable mixture.

7. In a separate bowl, prepare the flax eggs by mixing ground flaxseed with water. Let it sit for a few minutes until it thickens.

8. Pour the flax eggs over the bread and vegetables, tossing everything to coat evenly.

9. Gradually pour gluten-free vegetable broth over the mixture, stirring as you go. Add enough broth to moisten the stuffing to your desired consistency.

10. Transfer the gluten-free stuffing to the greased baking dish, spreading it evenly.

11. Cover the baking dish with aluminum foil and bake in the preheated oven for 30 minutes.

12. Remove the foil and bake for an additional 15-20 minutes or until the top is golden brown and crispy.

13. Garnish with chopped fresh parsley if desired.

Snack Ideas:

Guacamole with Gluten-Free Tortilla Chips:

Ingredients:

- 3 ripe avocados
- 1 small red onion, finely diced
- 1-2 tomatoes, diced
- 1 jalapeño, seeds removed and finely chopped
- 1/4 cup fresh cilantro, chopped

- 2 cloves garlic, minced
- Juice of 2 limes
- Salt and black pepper to taste

Instructions:

1. Cut the avocados in half, remove the pits, and scoop the flesh into a mixing bowl.
2. Mash the avocados using a fork or potato masher until you achieve your desired level of creaminess.
3. Add the finely diced red onion, diced tomatoes, chopped jalapeño, minced garlic, and chopped cilantro to the mashed avocados.
4. Squeeze the juice of two limes over the mixture.
5. Season with salt and black pepper to taste.
6. Gently fold all the ingredients together until well combined.
7. Taste and adjust the seasoning if needed.
8. Cover the guacamole with plastic wrap, ensuring the wrap is pressed directly onto the surface of the guacamole to prevent browning. Refrigerate until ready to serve.

Gluten-Free Tortilla Chips:

Ingredients:

- Gluten-free corn tortillas
- Olive oil
- Salt

Instructions:

1. Preheat your oven to 350°F (175°C).
2. Stack the gluten-free corn tortillas and cut them into wedges using a sharp knife or a pizza cutter.
3. Arrange the tortilla wedges on a baking sheet in a single layer.
4. Brush each wedge lightly with olive oil.
5. Sprinkle salt over the oiled tortilla wedges.
6. Bake in the preheated oven for 10-12 minutes or until the chips are golden brown and crispy.

7. Allow the gluten-free tortilla chips to cool before serving.

Trail Mix with Nuts and Dried Fruits:

Ingredients:

- 1 cup almonds
- 1 cup walnuts
- 1 cup cashews
- 1 cup pumpkin seeds
- 1 cup dried cranberries
- 1 cup raisins
- 1 cup dried apricots, chopped
- 1 cup dark chocolate chips or chunks

Instructions:

1. In a large mixing bowl, combine almonds, walnuts, cashews, pumpkin seeds, dried cranberries, raisins, dried apricots, and dark chocolate chips.
2. Mix all the ingredients together until well combined.
3. Store the trail mix in an airtight container to keep it fresh.
4. Customize the trail mix by adjusting the quantities of nuts, dried fruits, and chocolate chips according to your preferences.
5. Portion out the trail mix into snack-sized bags for convenient and healthy on-the-go snacks.

Crispy Chickpeas:

Ingredients:

- 2 cans (15 oz each) chickpeas (garbanzo beans), drained and rinsed
- 2 tablespoons olive oil
- 1 teaspoon smoked paprika
- 1 teaspoon ground cumin
- 1/2 teaspoon garlic powder

- 1/2 teaspoon onion powder
- 1/4 teaspoon cayenne pepper (adjust to taste)
- Salt to taste

Instructions:

1. Preheat your oven to 400°F (200°C).
2. Rinse and drain the canned chickpeas. Pat them dry with a clean kitchen towel to remove excess moisture.
3. In a large bowl, toss the chickpeas with olive oil, smoked paprika, ground cumin, garlic powder, onion powder, cayenne pepper, and salt until the chickpeas are evenly coated.
4. Spread the seasoned chickpeas in a single layer on a baking sheet lined with parchment paper.
5. Roast in the preheated oven for 25-30 minutes or until the chickpeas are golden brown and crispy. Shake the pan or stir the chickpeas halfway through the cooking time for even crispiness.
6. Remove from the oven and let the crispy chickpeas cool slightly.
7. Taste and adjust the seasoning if needed.

Fruit Kabobs:

Ingredients:

- Assorted fresh fruits (such as strawberries, grapes, pineapple, melon, kiwi, and berries)
- Wooden or metal skewers

Optional:

- Honey or maple syrup for drizzling
- Mint leaves for garnish

Instructions:

1. Wash and prepare the fresh fruits. If using pineapple or melon, cut them into bite-sized pieces.

2. Thread the assorted fruits onto the skewers in a colorful and appealing pattern.

3. Repeat the process until you have assembled all the fruit kabobs.

4. Optional: Drizzle honey or maple syrup over the fruit kabobs for a touch of sweetness.

5. Garnish with fresh mint leaves for added freshness.

6. Arrange the fruit kabobs on a serving platter or plate.

Homemade Popcorn:

Ingredients:

- 1/2 cup popcorn kernels
- 2 tablespoons vegetable oil
- Salt to taste
- Optional toppings: melted butter, nutritional yeast, grated cheese, cinnamon sugar, or your favorite seasoning

Instructions:

1. In a large, heavy-bottomed pot with a lid, heat the vegetable oil over medium heat.

2. Add three popcorn kernels to the pot and cover with the lid.

3. Once the test kernels pop, add the remaining popcorn kernels to the pot.

4. Cover the pot with the lid and shake it gently to distribute the heat.

5. Continue to shake the pot occasionally to prevent burning and ensure even popping.

6. When the popping slows down to a few seconds between pops, remove the pot from the heat.

7. Let the popcorn sit for a moment to allow any remaining kernels to pop.

8. Carefully remove the lid, keeping it away from your face to avoid steam.

9. Season the popcorn with salt and any desired toppings. Toss gently to coat.

Greek Yogurt Parfait with Berries:

Ingredients:

- 1 cup Greek yogurt

- 1 cup mixed berries (strawberries, blueberries, raspberries)

- 2 tablespoons honey or maple syrup

- 1/4 cup granola

- 1 tablespoon chia seeds (optional)

- Fresh mint leaves for garnish (optional)

Instructions:

1. In a serving glass or bowl, start with a layer of Greek yogurt.

2. Add a layer of mixed berries on top of the yogurt.

3. Drizzle honey or maple syrup over the berries.

4. Sprinkle a layer of granola over the berries.

5. Optionally, add a sprinkle of chia seeds for added texture and nutritional benefits.

6. Repeat the layers until you reach the top of the glass or bowl.

7. Garnish the Greek Yogurt Parfait with fresh mint leaves for a burst of freshness.

8. Serve immediately and enjoy.

Edamame with Sea Salt:

Ingredients:

- 2 cups frozen edamame in pods

- Sea salt to taste

Instructions:

1. Bring a pot of water to a boil and add a generous pinch of salt.

2. Add the frozen edamame pods to the boiling water.

3. Cook the edamame for 4-5 minutes or until they are tender but still have a slight bite.

4. Drain the edamame in a colander and let them cool for a minute.

5. Place the cooked edamame in a serving bowl.

6. Sprinkle sea salt over the edamame, tossing them gently to coat.

7. Serve the Edamame with Sea Salt as a tasty and nutritious snack.

Sliced Apple with Almond Butter:

Ingredients:

- **1 apple, sliced**
- 2 tablespoons almond butter

Instructions:

1. Wash and slice the apple into thin wedges or rounds.
2. Place the apple slices on a serving plate.
3. In a small bowl, scoop out the almond butter.
4. Dip each apple slice into the almond butter or spread the almond butter on the apple slices.
5. Arrange the Sliced Apple with Almond Butter on the plate.

Vegetable Sticks with Hummus:

Ingredients:

- **Assorted vegetables** (carrots, cucumber, bell peppers, celery, cherry tomatoes, etc.), cut into sticks or wedges
- Hummus for dipping

Instructions:

1. Wash and prepare the assorted vegetables by cutting them into stick or wedge shapes.
2. Arrange the vegetable sticks on a serving platter.
3. Place a bowl of hummus in the center of the platter for dipping.
4. Serve the Vegetable Sticks with Hummus as a colorful and nutritious appetizer or snack.

Energy Bites:

Ingredients:

- 1 cup rolled oats
- 1/2 cup nut butter (such as almond butter or peanut butter)

- 1/3 cup honey or maple syrup

- 1/2 cup ground flaxseed

- 1/2 cup chocolate chips or chopped nuts

- 1 teaspoon vanilla extract

- Pinch of salt (optional)

- Additional add-ins: chia seeds, shredded coconut, dried fruit, etc.

Instructions:

1. In a large bowl, combine rolled oats, nut butter, honey or maple syrup, ground flaxseed, chocolate chips or chopped nuts, vanilla extract, and a pinch of salt if desired.

2. Mix the ingredients until well combined.

3. If the mixture seems too wet, add more rolled oats. If it's too dry, add a bit more nut butter or honey.

4. Optionally, add in any additional ingredients like chia seeds, shredded coconut, or dried fruit.

5. Once the mixture reaches a dough-like consistency, refrigerate it for 15-30 minutes to make it easier to handle.

6. After refrigeration, use your hands to roll the mixture into bite-sized balls.

7. Place the Energy Bites on a parchment-lined tray or plate.

8. Refrigerate the energy bites for at least 30 minutes to firm up.

9. Once firm, transfer the energy bites to an airtight container and store them in the refrigerator.

Gluten-Free Rice Cakes with Avocado:

Ingredients:

- Gluten-free rice cakes

- 1 ripe avocado

- Lemon juice (from half a lemon)

- Salt and black pepper to taste

- Optional toppings: red pepper flakes, sesame seeds, or microgreens

Instructions:

1. Cut the avocado in half, remove the pit, and scoop the flesh into a bowl.

2. Mash the avocado with a fork and mix in the lemon juice to prevent browning.

3. Season the mashed avocado with salt and black pepper to taste. Adjust the seasoning if needed.

4. Spread the mashed avocado evenly onto gluten-free rice cakes.

5. Optionally, sprinkle red pepper flakes, sesame seeds, or top with microgreens for added flavor and texture.

6. Serve the Gluten-Free Rice Cakes with Avocado as a simple and wholesome snack or light meal.

CHAPTER 8: DESSERTS AND TREATS

Gluten-Free Chocolate Cake:

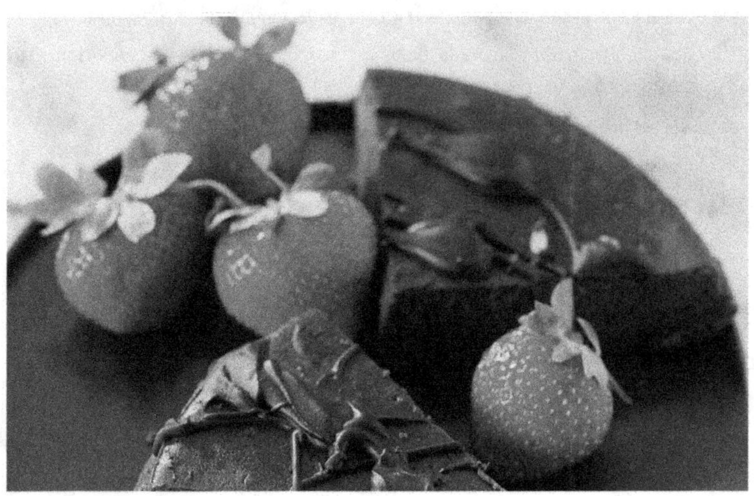

Ingredients:

- 1 cup gluten-free all-purpose flour
- 1/2 cup cocoa powder
- 1 teaspoon baking powder
- 1/2 teaspoon baking soda
- 1/2 teaspoon salt
- 1/2 cup unsalted butter, softened
- 1 cup granulated sugar
- 2 large eggs
- 1 teaspoon vanilla extract
- 1 cup buttermilk (or dairy-free alternative)

For Chocolate Ganache (optional):

- 1/2 cup heavy cream (or coconut cream for dairy-free)
- 1 cup semi-sweet chocolate chips

Instructions:

1. Preheat your oven to 350°F (175°C). Grease and flour a round cake pan.
2. In a medium bowl, whisk together gluten-free all-purpose flour, cocoa powder, baking powder, baking soda, and salt.
3. In a large bowl, using an electric mixer, cream together softened butter and granulated sugar until light and fluffy.
4. Add eggs one at a time, beating well after each addition. Add vanilla extract and mix until combined.
5. Gradually add the dry ingredients to the wet ingredients, alternating with buttermilk. Begin and end with the dry ingredients, mixing just until combined. Do not overmix.
6. Pour the batter into the prepared cake pan and smooth the top.
7. Bake in the preheated oven for 25-30 minutes or until a toothpick inserted into the center comes out clean.
8. Allow the cake to cool in the pan for 10 minutes, then transfer it to a wire rack to cool completely.
9. Optional: Prepare the chocolate ganache by heating the cream in a small saucepan until it begins to simmer. Remove from heat and pour over the chocolate chips in a heatproof bowl. Let it sit for a minute, then stir until smooth. Let the ganache cool for a few minutes before pouring it over the cooled cake.
10. Once the ganache is set, slice and serve the Gluten-Free.

Vegan Chocolate Avocado Mousse:

Ingredients:

- 2 ripe avocados
- 1/2 cup cocoa powder
- 1/2 cup maple syrup or agave nectar

- 1/4 cup coconut milk

- 1 teaspoon vanilla extract

- Pinch of salt

Instructions:

1. Peel and pit the avocados, placing the flesh in a blender or food processor.

2. Add cocoa powder, maple syrup (or agave nectar), coconut milk, vanilla extract, and a pinch of salt to the blender.

3. Blend the ingredients until smooth and creamy, scraping down the sides as needed.

4. Taste the mixture and adjust sweetness if necessary by adding more maple syrup or agave.

5. Once the mousse reaches a smooth consistency, transfer it to serving dishes or bowls.

6. Chill the mousse in the refrigerator for at least 2 hours before serving.

7. Garnish with berries, shredded coconut or chopped nuts if desired.

Almond Flour Lemon Bars:

Ingredients:

For the Crust:

- 1 1/2 cups almond flour

- 1/4 cup coconut flour

- 1/4 cup melted coconut oil

- 1/4 cup maple syrup

- 1/2 teaspoon vanilla extract

- 1/4 teaspoon salt

For the Lemon Filling:

- 1 cup fresh lemon juice (about 4-5 lemons)

- 1 tablespoon lemon zest

- 1/2 cup maple syrup

- 4 large eggs

- 1/4 cup almond flour
- 1/2 teaspoon baking powder
- Pinch of salt
- Powdered sugar for dusting (optional)

Instructions:

For the Crust:

1. Preheat the oven to 350°F (175°C) and line an 8x8-inch baking dish with parchment paper.
2. In a bowl, combine almond flour, coconut flour, melted coconut oil, maple syrup, vanilla extract, and salt. Mix until well combined.
3. Press the crust mixture into the bottom of the prepared baking dish, creating an even layer.
4. Bake the crust for 10-12 minutes or until it starts to turn golden. Remove from the oven and let it cool slightly.

For the Lemon Filling:

1. In a bowl, whisk together fresh lemon juice, lemon zest, maple syrup, eggs, almond flour, baking powder, and a pinch of salt until smooth.
2. Pour the lemon filling over the baked crust, spreading it evenly.
3. Bake for an additional 20-25 minutes or until the edges are set, and the center is slightly firm.
4. Allow the lemon bars to cool completely in the baking dish before placing them in the refrigerator to chill for at least 2 hours.
5. Once chilled, cut into squares, and dust with powdered sugar if desired.

Coconut Milk Rice Pudding:

Ingredients:

- 1 cup Arborio rice
- 4 cups coconut milk
- 1/2 cup sugar

- 1 teaspoon vanilla extract

- 1/2 teaspoon ground cinnamon

- 1/4 teaspoon salt

- Optional toppings: toasted coconut flakes, sliced almonds, or fresh fruit

Instructions:

1. Rinse the Arborio rice under cold water until the water runs clear.

2. In a medium-sized saucepan, combine the rinsed rice, coconut milk, sugar, vanilla extract, ground cinnamon, and salt.

3. Bring the mixture to a gentle boil over medium heat, stirring frequently to prevent the rice from sticking to the bottom of the pan.

4. Once it reaches a boil, reduce the heat to low and simmer uncovered. Continue stirring occasionally to ensure the rice cooks evenly.

5. Cook for about 25-30 minutes or until the rice is tender and the mixture has thickened to a creamy consistency.

6. If the rice pudding becomes too thick, you can add a bit more coconut milk to achieve your desired consistency.

7. Remove the saucepan from heat and let the rice pudding cool for a few minutes.

8. Serve the coconut milk rice pudding warm or chilled, and top with toasted coconut flakes, sliced almonds, or fresh fruit if desired.

Gluten-Free Apple Crisp:

Ingredients:

For the Filling:

- 6 cups peeled and sliced apples (such as Granny Smith or Honeycrisp)

- 1/4 cup maple syrup

- 2 tablespoons lemon juice

- 1 teaspoon ground cinnamon

- 1/4 teaspoon nutmeg

- 1 tablespoon gluten-free flour (e.g., almond flour or rice flour)

For the Topping:

- 1 cup gluten-free rolled oats
- 1/2 cup almond flour
- 1/4 cup chopped nuts (such as pecans or walnuts)
- 1/4 cup melted coconut oil or butter
- 1/4 cup maple syrup
- 1 teaspoon vanilla extract
- 1/4 teaspoon salt

Instructions:

1. Preheat your oven to 350°F (175°C) and grease a baking dish.
2. In a large bowl, combine the sliced apples, maple syrup, lemon juice, ground cinnamon, nutmeg, and gluten-free flour. Toss until the apples are evenly coated.
3. Transfer the apple mixture to the prepared baking dish, spreading it out evenly.

For the Topping:

1. In a separate bowl, combine gluten-free rolled oats, almond flour, chopped nuts, melted coconut oil or butter, maple syrup, vanilla extract, and salt. Mix until everything is well combined.
2. Sprinkle the topping evenly over the apple mixture in the baking dish.
3. Bake in the preheated oven for 35-40 minutes or until the topping is golden brown, and the apples are tender.
4. Remove from the oven and let it cool for a few minutes before serving.
5. Serve the gluten-free apple crisp warm, optionally with a scoop of vanilla ice cream or a dollop of whipped coconut cream.

Chia Seed Pudding with Berries:

Ingredients:

- 1/4 cup chia seeds
- 1 cup coconut milk (or any plant-based milk of your choice)
- 1 tablespoon maple syrup (adjust to taste)

- 1/2 teaspoon vanilla extract
- Mixed berries (strawberries, blueberries, raspberries) for topping

Instructions:

1. In a bowl, combine chia seeds, coconut milk, maple syrup, and vanilla extract.
2. Whisk the mixture well to ensure the chia seeds are evenly distributed. Let it sit for a few minutes.
3. Whisk again after a few minutes to prevent clumping, and then cover the bowl or transfer the mixture to individual jars.
4. Refrigerate the chia seed pudding for at least 2 hours or overnight, allowing it to thicken.
5. Before serving, give the pudding a good stir to achieve a creamy consistency.
6. Top the chia seed pudding with a generous amount of mixed berries.
7. Optionally, drizzle a bit more maple syrup on top for added sweetness.

Pumpkin Pie with Almond Flour Crust:

Ingredients:

For the Almond Flour Crust:

- 2 cups almond flour
- 1/4 cup melted coconut oil
- 2 tablespoons maple syrup
- 1/2 teaspoon cinnamon
- Pinch of salt

For the Pumpkin Pie Filling:

- 1 can (15 oz) pumpkin puree
- 3/4 cup coconut milk
- 1/2 cup maple syrup
- 2 large eggs
- 1 teaspoon vanilla extract
- 1 teaspoon ground cinnamon

- 1/2 teaspoon ground ginger
- 1/4 teaspoon ground nutmeg
- 1/4 teaspoon salt

Instructions:

For the Almond Flour Crust:

1. Preheat your oven to 350°F (175°C).
2. In a bowl, combine almond flour, melted coconut oil, maple syrup, cinnamon, and a pinch of salt.
3. Mix until a dough forms.
4. Press the dough into the bottom of a pie dish, covering the bottom and sides evenly.
5. Bake the crust for 10-12 minutes or until it's slightly golden. Remove from the oven and let it cool.

For the Pumpkin Pie Filling:

1. In a large bowl, whisk together pumpkin puree, coconut milk, maple syrup, eggs, vanilla extract, cinnamon, ginger, nutmeg, and salt until well combined.
2. Pour the pumpkin filling into the pre-baked almond flour crust.
3. Bake in the preheated oven for 40-45 minutes or until the center is set.
4. Allow the pumpkin pie to cool completely before refrigerating for at least 2 hours to set.
5. Once chilled, slice and serve.
6. Optionally, top with whipped coconut cream or a sprinkle of cinnamon.

Vegan Chocolate Chip Cookies:

Ingredients:

- 1/2 cup coconut oil, melted
- 1/2 cup brown sugar, packed
- 1/4 cup granulated sugar
- 1/4 cup unsweetened applesauce

- 1 teaspoon vanilla extract
- 2 cups all-purpose flour
- 1/2 teaspoon baking soda
- 1/2 teaspoon salt
- 1 cup vegan chocolate chips

Instructions:

1. Preheat your oven to 350°F (175°C) and line a baking sheet with parchment paper.
2. In a large bowl, whisk together melted coconut oil, brown sugar, granulated sugar, applesauce, and vanilla extract until well combined.
3. In a separate bowl, whisk together the flour, baking soda, and salt.
4. Gradually add the dry ingredients to the wet ingredients, mixing until just combined.
5. Fold in the vegan chocolate chips until evenly distributed throughout the cookie dough.
6. Using a cookie scoop or spoon, drop rounded tablespoons of dough onto the prepared baking sheet, spacing them about 2 inches apart.
7. Bake in the preheated oven for 10-12 minutes or until the edges are golden brown.
8. Allow the cookies to cool on the baking sheet for a few minutes before transferring them to a wire rack to cool completely.

Gluten-Free Cheesecake Bites:

Ingredients:

For the Crust:

- 1 1/2 cups gluten-free graham cracker crumbs (or almond flour for a nuttier option)
- 1/4 cup melted coconut oil
- 2 tablespoons maple syrup
- Pinch of salt

For the Cheesecake Filling:

* 2 cups dairy-free cream cheese (such as vegan cream cheese)

* 1/2 cup coconut sugar (or sweetener of your choice)

* 2 teaspoons vanilla extract

* 2 tablespoons lemon juice

* 2 tablespoons cornstarch or arrowroot powder

* Pinch of salt

Instructions:

For the Crust:

1. Preheat your oven to 325°F (163°C) and line a mini muffin tin with paper liners.

2. In a bowl, combine gluten-free graham cracker crumbs, melted coconut oil, maple syrup, and a pinch of salt. Mix until the crumbs are well-coated.

3. Press about a tablespoon of the crust mixture into the bottom of each mini muffin cup, creating a firm base.

4. Bake the crusts in the preheated oven for 8-10 minutes or until they become golden. Remove from the oven and let them cool.

For the Cheesecake Filling:

1. In a mixing bowl, beat the dairy-free cream cheese until smooth and creamy.

2. Add coconut sugar, vanilla extract, lemon juice, cornstarch or arrowroot powder, and a pinch of salt. Mix until well combined.

3. Spoon or pipe the cheesecake filling onto the cooled crusts in the mini muffin tin.

4. Refrigerate the cheesecake bites for at least 2-3 hours or until set.

5. Once set, remove the cheesecake bites from the muffin tin and serve.

Mixed Berry Sorbet:

Ingredients:

* 3 cups mixed berries (strawberries, blueberries, raspberries, blackberries)

* 1/2 cup granulated sugar (adjust to taste)

* 1 tablespoon fresh lemon juice

* 1/2 cup water

Instructions:

1. Wash the berries thoroughly and remove any stems.
2. In a blender or food processor, combine the mixed berries, granulated sugar, fresh lemon juice, and water.
3. Blend the mixture until it becomes a smooth puree.
4. Taste the mixture and adjust the sweetness by adding more sugar if needed.
5. Strain the puree through a fine-mesh sieve into a bowl to remove seeds and pulp. Press down with a spoon to extract as much liquid as possible.
6. Pour the strained mixture into a shallow dish, spreading it evenly.
7. Place the dish in the freezer and let it freeze for about 2 hours.
8. After 2 hours, take the sorbet out and scrape it with a fork to break up any ice crystals. Repeat this process every hour for the next 2-3 hours.
9. Once the sorbet has a smooth, slushy consistency, transfer it into a sealed container and freeze for an additional 2-4 hours or until firm.
10. Before serving, let the sorbet sit at room temperature for a few minutes to soften slightly.
11. Scoop the Mixed Berry Sorbet into bowls or cones and enjoy the refreshing treat!

Chocolate-Dipped Strawberries:

Ingredients:

- Fresh strawberries, washed and dried
- 6 ounces dark chocolate, chopped (or vegan chocolate for a dairy-free option)
- 1 tablespoon coconut oil (optional, for smoother dipping)
- Toppings (optional): chopped nuts, shredded coconut, sprinkles

Instructions:

1. Line a tray or plate with parchment paper.
2. In a heatproof bowl, melt the dark chocolate in the microwave or using a double boiler. If using coconut oil, add it to the chocolate while melting for smoother dipping.

3. Hold each strawberry by the stem and dip it into the melted chocolate, swirling to coat about two-thirds of the strawberry.

4. Allow excess chocolate to drip back into the bowl.

5. Optional: Roll the dipped strawberry in your choice of toppings, such as chopped nuts, shredded coconut, or sprinkles.

6. Place the dipped strawberries on the prepared tray or plate.

7. Repeat the dipping process with the remaining strawberries.

8. Place the tray in the refrigerator for about 15-20 minutes to let the chocolate set.

9. Once the chocolate is firm, transfer the chocolate-dipped strawberries to a serving plate.

10. Serve and enjoy these delicious Chocolate-Dipped Strawberries as a sweet treat or dessert!

Treat Ideas:

Gluten-Free Brownie Bites:

Ingredients:
- 1 cup almond flour
- 1/2 cup cocoa powder
- 1/2 cup coconut sugar
- 1/4 teaspoon baking soda
- 1/4 teaspoon salt
- 1/4 cup coconut oil, melted
- 2 large eggs
- 1 teaspoon vanilla extract
- 1/2 cup dark chocolate chips

Instructions:
1. Preheat your oven to 350°F (175°C) and grease a mini muffin tin.

2. In a bowl, whisk together almond flour, cocoa powder, coconut sugar, baking soda, and salt.

3. In another bowl, whisk together melted coconut oil, eggs, and vanilla extract until well combined.

4. Add the wet ingredients to the dry ingredients and mix until just combined.

5. Fold in the dark chocolate chips.

6. Using a tablespoon or cookie scoop, fill each mini muffin cup with the brownie batter.

7. Bake in the preheated oven for 10-12 minutes or until a toothpick inserted into the center comes out with moist crumbs (not wet batter).

8. Allow the brownie bites to cool in the muffin tin for a few minutes before transferring them to a wire rack to cool completely.

9. Once cooled, serve and enjoy your Gluten-Free Brownie Bites!

Trail Mix Energy Bars:

Ingredients:

- 1 cup old-fashioned oats
- 1/2 cup unsweetened shredded coconut
- 1/2 cup chopped nuts (almonds, walnuts, or your choice)
- 1/4 cup seeds (pumpkin seeds, sunflower seeds)
- 1/4 cup dried fruit (raisins, cranberries, apricots), chopped if large
- 1/4 cup mini chocolate chips (optional)
- 1/2 cup nut butter (almond butter, peanut butter, or a mix)
- 1/4 cup honey or maple syrup
- 1 teaspoon vanilla extract
- Pinch of salt

Instructions:

1. Preheat your oven to 350°F (175°C). Line a baking dish with parchment paper, leaving some overhang for easy removal.

2. In a large mixing bowl, combine oats, shredded coconut, chopped nuts, seeds, dried fruit, and mini chocolate chips if using.

3. In a small saucepan, heat nut butter, honey (or maple syrup), vanilla extract, and a pinch of salt over low heat. Stir until well combined and smooth.

4. Pour the wet mixture over the dry ingredients and mix until everything is evenly coated.

5. Transfer the mixture to the prepared baking dish and press it down firmly to create an even layer.

6. Bake in the preheated oven for 15-18 minutes or until the edges turn golden brown.

7. Allow the bars to cool completely in the baking dish.

8. Once cooled, lift the parchment paper to easily remove the bars from the dish and place them on a cutting board.

9. Cut into bars or squares of your desired size.

10. Store the Trail Mix Energy Bars in an airtight container at room temperature or refrigerate for longer shelf life.

No-Bake Almond Butter Energy Balls:

Ingredients:

- 1 cup old-fashioned oats
- 1/2 cup almond butter
- 1/3 cup honey or maple syrup
- 1/2 cup ground flaxseed
- 1/2 cup shredded coconut (unsweetened)
- 1 teaspoon vanilla extract
- Pinch of salt
- Optional: 1/3 cup mini chocolate chips or chopped nuts for extra texture

Instructions:

1. In a large mixing bowl, combine old-fashioned oats, almond butter, honey (or maple syrup), ground flaxseed, shredded coconut, vanilla extract, and a pinch of salt.
2. If using, add mini chocolate chips or chopped nuts to the mixture.
3. Stir the ingredients until well combined. If the mixture seems too dry, you can add a bit more almond butter or honey to achieve the right consistency.
4. Place the bowl in the refrigerator for about 15-30 minutes. Chilling makes it easier to form the mixture into balls.
5. Once chilled, take small portions of the mixture and roll them into bite-sized balls using your hands.
6. Arrange the almond butter energy balls on a parchment-lined tray or plate.
7. Place the tray in the refrigerator for at least 30 minutes to allow the energy balls to firm up.
8. Once firm, transfer the energy balls to an airtight container and store in the refrigerator.

Gluten-Free Chocolate Covered Pretzels:

Ingredients:

- Gluten-free pretzels
- 8 ounces gluten-free chocolate (dark, milk, or white chocolate)
- 1 tablespoon coconut oil (optional, for smoother chocolate)
- Toppings (optional): chopped nuts, shredded coconut, sprinkles

Instructions:

1. Line a tray or baking sheet with parchment paper.
2. In a microwave-safe bowl or using a double boiler, melt the gluten-free chocolate. If using coconut oil, mix it with the chocolate for smoother dipping.
3. Stir the melted chocolate until it's smooth and well combined.
4. Hold each pretzel by its end and dip it into the melted chocolate, coating about half or two-thirds of the pretzel.

5. Allow excess chocolate to drip back into the bowl.

6. Optional: Sprinkle or roll the chocolate-covered part of the pretzel in your choice of toppings, such as chopped nuts or shredded coconut.

7. Place the chocolate-covered pretzels on the prepared tray.

8. Repeat the dipping process with the remaining pretzels.

9. Allow the chocolate-covered pretzels to set by placing them in the refrigerator for about 15-20 minutes.

10. Once the chocolate is firm, transfer the pretzels to a serving plate.

Vegan Rice Krispie Treats:

Ingredients:

- 6 cups vegan rice cereal (make sure it's gluten-free if needed)
- 4 cups vegan marshmallows
- 1/4 cup vegan butter or coconut oil
- 1/2 teaspoon vanilla extract
- Pinch of salt

Instructions:

1. Grease a 9x13-inch baking dish or line it with parchment paper.

2. In a large pot over low heat, melt the vegan butter or coconut oil.

3. Add the vegan marshmallows to the pot and stir continuously until they are completely melted and smooth.

4. Remove the pot from the heat and stir in the vanilla extract and a pinch of salt.

5. Quickly add the vegan rice cereal to the marshmallow mixture. Stir until the cereal is evenly coated.

6. Transfer the mixture to the prepared baking dish and press it down firmly with a spatula or your hands to create an even layer.

7. Allow the vegan rice krispie treats to cool and set for at least 30 minutes.

8. Once cooled, cut the treats into squares or bars.

Maple Cinnamon Roasted Almonds:

Ingredients:

- 2 cups raw almonds
- 2 tablespoons maple syrup
- 1 tablespoon coconut oil, melted
- 1 teaspoon ground cinnamon
- 1/4 teaspoon salt

Instructions:

1. Preheat your oven to 325°F (163°C). Line a baking sheet with parchment paper.
2. In a bowl, mix together raw almonds, maple syrup, melted coconut oil, ground cinnamon, and salt. Ensure the almonds are evenly coated.
3. Spread the almond mixture in a single layer on the prepared baking sheet.
4. Bake in the preheated oven for 20-25 minutes, stirring halfway through to ensure even roasting.
5. Keep a close eye on the almonds in the last few minutes to prevent burning.
6. Once the almonds are golden brown and fragrant, remove them from the oven.
7. Let the maple cinnamon roasted almonds cool completely on the baking sheet. They will continue to crisp up as they cool.
8. Once cooled, break apart any almonds that may have stuck together.
9. Store in an airtight container at room temperature.

Coconut Bliss Balls:

Ingredients:

- 1 cup shredded coconut (plus extra for coating)
- 1 cup pitted dates, softened
- 1/4 cup coconut oil, melted
- 2 tablespoons maple syrup or agave nectar
- 1 teaspoon vanilla extract
- Pinch of salt

Instructions:

1. In a food processor, combine shredded coconut, softened dates, melted coconut oil, maple syrup (or agave nectar), vanilla extract, and a pinch of salt.
2. Process the mixture until it forms a sticky, uniform dough.
3. If the mixture is too dry, you can add a little more melted coconut oil or a splash of water to help bind it together.
4. Scoop out small portions of the mixture and roll them into bite-sized balls using your hands.
5. Roll each bliss ball in additional shredded coconut to coat them evenly.
6. Place the coconut bliss balls on a parchment-lined tray or plate.
7. Refrigerate the bliss balls for at least 30 minutes to allow them to firm up.
8. Once chilled, transfer the coconut bliss balls to an airtight container and store in the refrigerator.

Gluten-Free Oatmeal Cookies:

Ingredients:

- 1 cup gluten-free rolled oats
- 3/4 cup almond flour
- 1/2 teaspoon baking soda
- 1/4 teaspoon salt
- 1/2 teaspoon ground cinnamon
- 1/4 cup coconut oil, melted
- 1/4 cup maple syrup or honey
- 1 large egg
- 1 teaspoon vanilla extract
- 1/2 cup raisins or chocolate chips (optional)

Instructions:

1. Preheat your oven to 350°F (175°C). Line a baking sheet with parchment paper.

2. In a bowl, mix together gluten-free rolled oats, almond flour, baking soda, salt, and ground cinnamon.

3. In another bowl, whisk together melted coconut oil, maple syrup (or honey), egg, and vanilla extract until well combined.

4. Add the wet ingredients to the dry ingredients and mix until a cookie dough forms.

5. If desired, fold in raisins or chocolate chips.

6. Drop rounded tablespoons of dough onto the prepared baking sheet, spacing them about 2 inches apart.

7. Flatten each cookie slightly with the back of a spoon or your hand.

8. Bake in the preheated oven for 10-12 minutes or until the edges are golden brown.

9. Allow the gluten-free oatmeal cookies to cool on the baking sheet for a few minutes before transferring them to a wire rack to cool completely.

10. Once cooled, store in an airtight container.

Chocolate Coconut Chia Pudding Parfait:

Ingredients:

For the Chocolate Coconut Chia Pudding:

- 1/4 cup chia seeds
- 1 cup coconut milk
- 2 tablespoons cocoa powder
- 2-3 tablespoons maple syrup or agave nectar
- 1/2 teaspoon vanilla extract
- Pinch of salt

For the Parfait:

- Chocolate Coconut Chia Pudding
- 1/2 cup coconut yogurt (or any non-dairy yogurt)
- 1/4 cup shredded coconut (toasted, optional)
- Fresh berries for topping

Instructions:

For the Chocolate Coconut Chia Pudding:

1. In a bowl, whisk together chia seeds, coconut milk, cocoa powder, maple syrup (or agave nectar), vanilla extract, and a pinch of salt.
2. Whisk thoroughly to ensure there are no lumps and the cocoa powder is well incorporated.
3. Let the mixture sit for a few minutes, then whisk again to avoid clumping.
4. Cover the bowl and refrigerate the chia pudding for at least 2 hours or overnight to allow it to thicken.

For the Parfait:

1. Once the Chocolate Coconut Chia Pudding has set, layer it in serving glasses or jars with coconut yogurt.
2. Repeat the layers until you fill the glasses or jars.
3. Top the parfait with fresh berries and shredded coconut.
4. Optionally, toast the shredded coconut in a dry pan over medium heat until golden brown for added flavor.
5. Serve immediately or refrigerate until ready to enjoy.

Frozen Banana Pops:

Ingredients:

- Bananas, peeled and cut in half
- Wooden popsicle sticks
- 1 cup dark chocolate chips (or vegan chocolate chips)
- 2 tablespoons coconut oil
- Toppings (optional): chopped nuts, shredded coconut, sprinkles

Instructions:

1. Insert a wooden popsicle stick into each banana half, leaving enough exposed for holding.
2. Place the bananas on a parchment-lined tray and freeze them for at least 2 hours or until solid.

3. In a microwave-safe bowl or using a double boiler, melt the dark chocolate chips with coconut oil. Stir until smooth.

4. Remove the frozen bananas from the freezer.

5. Dip each banana into the melted chocolate, swirling to coat evenly.

6. Allow excess chocolate to drip back into the bowl.

7. Optional: Roll the chocolate-covered banana in your choice of toppings, such as chopped nuts or shredded coconut.

8. Place the chocolate-covered banana pops back on the parchment-lined tray.

9. Repeat the dipping process with the remaining bananas.

10. Place the tray back in the freezer for about 30 minutes or until the chocolate is set.

11. Once the chocolate is firm, transfer the frozen banana pops to a freezer-safe container for storage.

Vegan Peanut Butter Cups:

Ingredients:

- 1 cup vegan chocolate chips
- 2 tablespoons coconut oil
- 1/2 cup creamy peanut butter (or any nut or seed butter)
- 2 tablespoons powdered sugar (optional, for sweetening the peanut butter)
- 1/2 teaspoon vanilla extract
- Pinch of salt

Instructions:

1. Line a mini muffin tin with paper liners.

2. In a microwave-safe bowl or using a double boiler, melt the vegan chocolate chips with coconut oil. Stir until smooth.

3. Spoon a small amount of the melted chocolate into the bottom of each muffin cup, spreading it to coat the bottom and slightly up the sides.

4. Place the muffin tin in the freezer for about 10 minutes to set the chocolate.

5. In a separate bowl, mix together peanut butter, powdered sugar (if using), vanilla extract, and a pinch of salt until well combined.

6. Take the muffin tin out of the freezer and spoon a small amount of the peanut butter mixture into each cup, pressing it down slightly.

7. Pour the remaining melted chocolate over the peanut butter, covering it completely.

8. Optionally, sprinkle a pinch of salt on top of each peanut butter cup.

9. Place the muffin tin back in the freezer for about 30 minutes or until the peanut butter cups are firm.

10. Once firm, remove the vegan peanut butter cups from the muffin tin.

11. Store in the refrigerator or freezer until ready to serve.

CHAPTER 9: GLUTEN-FREE WEEKLY MEAL PLAN

Monday:

Breakfast: Quinoa Breakfast Bowl with Fresh Berries and Almond Milk

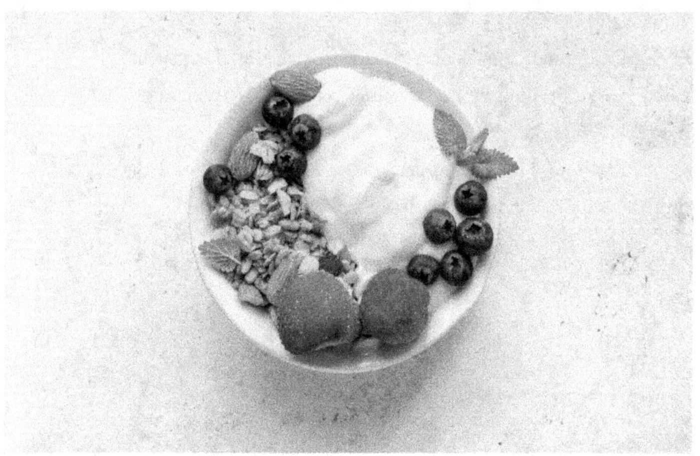

Ingredients:

- 1 cup cooked quinoa (prepared according to package instructions)
- 1/2 cup fresh mixed berries (strawberries, blueberries, raspberries)
- 1/4 cup almond milk (or any plant-based milk)
- 1 tablespoon maple syrup or agave nectar
- 1 tablespoon chopped nuts (almonds, walnuts)
- 1 teaspoon chia seeds (optional)
- 1/2 teaspoon vanilla extract
- Pinch of cinnamon (optional)

Instructions:

1. Cook quinoa according to package instructions. Fluff it with a fork and let it cool slightly.

2. In a bowl, combine the cooked quinoa with almond milk, maple syrup (or agave nectar), vanilla extract, and a pinch of cinnamon if desired.

3. Mix the ingredients well until the quinoa is evenly coated.

4. Transfer the quinoa mixture to a serving bowl.

5. Top the quinoa with fresh mixed berries, chopped nuts, and chia seeds.

6. Drizzle a bit more almond milk over the top.

7. Optionally, garnish with additional berries or a sprinkle of nuts for extra texture.

8. Serve and enjoy your wholesome Quinoa Breakfast Bowl with Fresh Berries and Almond Milk!

Lunch: Greek Chickpea Salad with Lemon Vinaigrette

Ingredients:

For the Salad:

- 1 can (15 oz) chickpeas, drained and rinsed
- 1 cup cherry tomatoes, halved
- 1 cucumber, diced
- 1/2 red onion, finely chopped
- 1/2 cup Kalamata olives, pitted and sliced
- 1/2 cup crumbled vegan feta cheese (optional)

For the Lemon Vinaigrette:

- 1/4 cup extra-virgin olive oil
- 2 tablespoons fresh lemon juice
- 1 teaspoon Dijon mustard
- 1 clove garlic, minced
- 1 teaspoon dried oregano

- Salt and pepper to taste

Instructions:

1. In a large bowl, combine chickpeas, cherry tomatoes, cucumber, red onion, Kalamata olives, and vegan feta cheese if using.
2. In a small bowl or jar, whisk together extra-virgin olive oil, fresh lemon juice, Dijon mustard, minced garlic, dried oregano, salt, and pepper. Adjust seasoning to taste.
3. Pour the lemon vinaigrette over the salad ingredients.
4. Toss the salad gently to ensure all ingredients are well coated with the vinaigrette.
5. Let the Greek Chickpea Salad marinate in the refrigerator for at least 15-30 minutes to allow the flavors to meld.
6. Before serving, give the salad a final toss and adjust the seasoning if necessary.
7. Serve as a refreshing and satisfying lunch, or as a side dish to complement your main course.

Dinner: Grilled Lemon Garlic Shrimp with Quinoa and Roasted Vegetables

Ingredients:

For the Grilled Lemon Garlic Shrimp:

- 1 pound large shrimp, peeled and deveined
- 2 tablespoons olive oil
- 3 cloves garlic, minced
- Zest and juice of 1 lemon
- 1 teaspoon dried oregano
- Salt and pepper to taste

For the Quinoa:

- 1 cup quinoa, rinsed
- 2 cups vegetable broth or water
- Salt to taste

For the Roasted Vegetables:

- 2 cups mixed vegetables (bell peppers, zucchini, cherry tomatoes)
- 2 tablespoons olive oil
- Salt and pepper to taste

Instructions:

For the Grilled Lemon Garlic Shrimp:

1. In a bowl, combine olive oil, minced garlic, lemon zest, lemon juice, dried oregano, salt, and pepper.
2. Add the peeled and deveined shrimp to the marinade. Toss to coat the shrimp evenly. Let it marinate for at least 15-30 minutes.
3. Preheat the grill to medium-high heat.
4. Thread the marinated shrimp onto skewers.
5. Grill the shrimp for 2-3 minutes per side or until they are opaque and cooked through.

For the Quinoa:

1. In a saucepan, combine quinoa and vegetable broth (or water). Add a pinch of salt.
2. Bring the mixture to a boil, then reduce the heat to low, cover, and simmer for 15-20 minutes or until the quinoa is cooked and liquid is absorbed.
3. Fluff the quinoa with a fork.

For the Roasted Vegetables:

1. Preheat the oven to 400°F (200°C).
2. In a bowl, toss the mixed vegetables with olive oil, salt, and pepper.
3. Spread the vegetables on a baking sheet in a single layer.
4. Roast in the preheated oven for 20-25 minutes or until the vegetables are tender and slightly caramelized.

Assembling the Dish:

1. Serve the grilled lemon garlic shrimp on a bed of cooked quinoa.
2. Arrange the roasted vegetables on the side.
3. Garnish with fresh herbs like parsley or dill.

Tuesday:

Breakfast: Vegan Smoothie Bowl with Mixed Berries and Almond Butter

Ingredients:

For the Smoothie Bowl:

- 1 cup frozen mixed berries (strawberries, blueberries, raspberries)
- 1 ripe banana, frozen
- 1/2 cup almond milk (or any plant-based milk)
- 1 tablespoon almond butter
- 1 tablespoon chia seeds (optional, for added texture)
- 1-2 tablespoons maple syrup or agave nectar (optional, for sweetness)

Toppings:

- Fresh berries (blueberries, strawberries, raspberries)
- Sliced banana
- Granola
- Drizzle of almond butter
- Chopped nuts (almonds, walnuts)

Instructions:

1. In a blender, combine frozen mixed berries, frozen banana, almond milk, almond butter, chia seeds (if using), and maple syrup or agave nectar.
2. Blend until smooth and creamy. Adjust the consistency by adding more almond milk if needed.
3. Pour the smoothie into a bowl.
4. Arrange your desired toppings on the smoothie bowl, such as fresh berries, sliced banana, granola, a drizzle of almond butter, and chopped nuts.
5. Customize the toppings to your liking, and get creative with the arrangement.
6. Enjoy your vibrant and nutritious Vegan Smoothie Bowl with Mixed Berries and Almond Butter for a delicious and energizing breakfast!

Lunch: Caprese Portobello Mushrooms with Balsamic Glaze

Ingredients:

For the Caprese Portobello Mushrooms:

- 4 large Portobello mushrooms, cleaned and stems removed
- 1 cup cherry tomatoes, halved
- 1 cup fresh mozzarella, sliced
- Fresh basil leaves
- 2 tablespoons olive oil
- Salt and black pepper to taste

For the Balsamic Glaze:

- 1/2 cup balsamic vinegar
- 2 tablespoons maple syrup or honey (optional, for sweetness)

Instructions:

For the Caprese Portobello Mushrooms:

1. Preheat the oven to 400°F (200°C).
2. Brush both sides of the Portobello mushrooms with olive oil and season with salt and black pepper.
3. Place the mushrooms on a baking sheet, gill side up.
4. In each mushroom cap, layer fresh mozzarella, cherry tomatoes, and fresh basil leaves.
5. Bake in the preheated oven for 15-20 minutes or until the mushrooms are tender and the cheese is melted and bubbly.

For the Balsamic Glaze:

1. In a small saucepan, combine balsamic vinegar and maple syrup or honey (if using).
2. Bring the mixture to a simmer over medium heat.
3. Reduce the heat to low and simmer for about 10-15 minutes or until the glaze thickens and coats the back of a spoon.
4. Remove from heat and let it cool slightly.

Assembling the Dish:

1. Drizzle the balsamic glaze over the Caprese Portobello Mushrooms.
2. Optionally, garnish with additional fresh basil leaves.
3. Serve the mushrooms warm.

Dinner: Vegan Lentil Soup with Gluten-Free Garlic Bread

For Vegan Lentil Soup:

Ingredients:

- 1 cup dried green or brown lentils, rinsed and drained
- 1 onion, diced
- 2 carrots, peeled and diced
- 2 celery stalks, diced
- 3 cloves garlic, minced
- 1 can (14 oz) diced tomatoes
- 6 cups vegetable broth
- 1 teaspoon ground cumin
- 1 teaspoon ground coriander
- 1 teaspoon smoked paprika
- 1/2 teaspoon turmeric
- Salt and black pepper to taste
- 2 cups chopped greens (spinach, kale, or Swiss chard)
- Fresh lemon juice (optional, for serving)

Instructions:

1. In a large pot, sauté the diced onion, carrots, and celery in a bit of olive oil until softened.
2. Add the minced garlic and sauté for another minute until fragrant.
3. Stir in the lentils, diced tomatoes, vegetable broth, ground cumin, ground coriander, smoked paprika, turmeric, salt, and black pepper.

4. Bring the soup to a boil, then reduce the heat to simmer. Cover and let it cook for about 20-25 minutes or until the lentils are tender.

5. Add the chopped greens and cook for an additional 5 minutes or until they are wilted.

6. Adjust the seasoning and add fresh lemon juice if desired.

7. Serve the vegan lentil soup hot.

For Gluten-Free Garlic Bread:

Ingredients:

- 1 loaf gluten-free bread
- 1/2 cup vegan butter, softened
- 4 cloves garlic, minced
- 2 tablespoons chopped fresh parsley
- Salt to taste

Instructions:

1. Preheat the oven to the temperature recommended on the gluten-free bread packaging.

2. In a bowl, mix together softened vegan butter, minced garlic, chopped fresh parsley, and salt.

3. Slice the gluten-free bread into individual slices.

4. Spread the garlic butter mixture over each slice.

5. Place the slices on a baking sheet and bake in the preheated oven according to the bread package instructions or until the edges are golden.

6. Serve the warm gluten-free garlic bread alongside the vegan lentil soup.

Wednesday:

Breakfast: Gluten-Free Oatmeal with Sliced Banana and Chia Seeds

Ingredients:

- 1/2 cup gluten-free rolled oats

- 1 cup almond milk (or any plant-based milk)
- 1 ripe banana, sliced
- 1 tablespoon chia seeds
- 1 tablespoon maple syrup or honey (optional, for sweetness)
- 1/4 teaspoon vanilla extract
- Pinch of salt
- Toppings: sliced banana, chia seeds, nuts, or a drizzle of nut butter (optional)

Instructions:

1. In a saucepan, combine gluten-free rolled oats and almond milk.
2. Place the saucepan over medium heat and bring the mixture to a simmer.
3. Reduce the heat to low and cook the oats, stirring occasionally, for about 5-7 minutes or until they reach your desired consistency.
4. Stir in sliced banana, chia seeds, maple syrup or honey (if using), vanilla extract, and a pinch of salt.
5. Continue to cook for an additional 2-3 minutes until the banana is softened, and chia seeds are well incorporated.
6. Remove the saucepan from heat.
7. Transfer the gluten-free oatmeal to a bowl.
8. Top the oatmeal with additional sliced banana, chia seeds, nuts, or a drizzle of nut butter if desired.
9. Serve the warm and nutritious Gluten-Free Oatmeal with Sliced Banana and Chia Seeds for a delightful breakfast!

Lunch: Stuffed Bell Peppers with Quinoa and Black Beans

Ingredients:

- 4 large bell peppers, halved and seeds removed
- 1 cup quinoa, rinsed
- 2 cups vegetable broth or water
- 1 can (15 oz) black beans, drained and rinsed

- 1 cup corn kernels (fresh, frozen, or canned)
- 1 cup diced tomatoes
- 1 cup diced red onion
- 2 cloves garlic, minced
- 1 teaspoon ground cumin
- 1 teaspoon chili powder
- Salt and black pepper to taste
- 1 cup shredded vegan cheese (optional)
- Fresh cilantro or parsley for garnish

Instructions:

1. Preheat the oven to 375°F (190°C).
2. In a saucepan, combine quinoa and vegetable broth (or water). Bring to a boil, then reduce the heat, cover, and simmer for 15-20 minutes or until quinoa is cooked and liquid is absorbed.
3. In a large mixing bowl, combine cooked quinoa, black beans, corn, diced tomatoes, diced red onion, minced garlic, ground cumin, chili powder, salt, and black pepper. Mix well.
4. Place the bell pepper halves in a baking dish.
5. Spoon the quinoa and black bean mixture into each bell pepper half, pressing down gently.
6. If using vegan cheese, sprinkle it over the stuffed peppers.
7. Cover the baking dish with foil and bake in the preheated oven for 25-30 minutes or until the peppers are tender.
8. Remove the foil and bake for an additional 5-10 minutes or until the cheese is melted and bubbly.
9. Garnish with fresh cilantro or parsley.
10. Serve the Stuffed Bell Peppers with Quinoa and Black Beans hot.

Dinner: Teriyaki Salmon with Stir-Fried Vegetables and Brown Rice

For Teriyaki Salmon:

Ingredients:

- 4 salmon fillets
- 1/4 cup soy sauce or tamari (gluten-free if needed)
- 2 tablespoons rice vinegar
- 2 tablespoons honey or maple syrup
- 1 tablespoon sesame oil
- 2 cloves garlic, minced
- 1 teaspoon grated ginger
- 2 tablespoons chopped green onions (for garnish)

Instructions:

1. In a bowl, whisk together soy sauce, rice vinegar, honey (or maple syrup), sesame oil, minced garlic, and grated ginger to create the teriyaki sauce.
2. Place the salmon fillets in a shallow dish and pour half of the teriyaki sauce over them. Marinate for at least 15-30 minutes.
3. Preheat the oven to 400°F (200°C).
4. Transfer the marinated salmon fillets to a baking sheet lined with parchment paper.
5. Bake in the preheated oven for 15-20 minutes or until the salmon is cooked through and flakes easily with a fork.
6. While the salmon is baking, heat the remaining teriyaki sauce in a small saucepan over low heat until it thickens slightly.
7. Once the salmon is done, brush it with the thickened teriyaki sauce and garnish with chopped green onions.

For Stir-Fried Vegetables:

Ingredients:

- 2 cups mixed vegetables (broccoli, bell peppers, carrots, snap peas)
- 1 tablespoon vegetable oil
- 1 tablespoon soy sauce or tamari

- 1 teaspoon sesame oil
- Sesame seeds for garnish (optional)

Instructions:

1. Heat vegetable oil in a wok or large skillet over medium-high heat.
2. Add mixed vegetables and stir-fry for 3-5 minutes or until they are crisp-tender.
3. Drizzle soy sauce and sesame oil over the vegetables. Toss to combine.
4. Garnish with sesame seeds if desired.

For Brown Rice:

Ingredients:

- 2 cups cooked brown rice

Instructions:

1. Cook brown rice according to package instructions.
2. Fluff the rice with a fork.

Assembling the Dish:

1. Serve the Teriyaki Salmon on a bed of brown rice.
2. Arrange the Stir-Fried Vegetables on the side.
3. Drizzle extra teriyaki sauce over the salmon if desired.
4. Enjoy your delicious and balanced Teriyaki Salmon with Stir-Fried Vegetables and Brown Rice for dinner!

Thursday:

Breakfast: Spinach and Feta Omelette with Avocado Slices

Ingredients:

- 3 large eggs
- 1 cup fresh spinach, chopped
- 1/4 cup feta cheese, crumbled
- Salt and black pepper to taste
- 1 tablespoon olive oil or butter

- 1/2 avocado, sliced

Instructions:

1. Crack the eggs into a bowl, season with salt and black pepper, and whisk until well beaten.
2. Heat olive oil or butter in a non-stick skillet over medium heat.
3. Add chopped spinach to the skillet and sauté for 1-2 minutes until wilted.
4. Pour the beaten eggs over the spinach in the skillet.
5. Allow the eggs to set slightly at the edges, then gently lift them with a spatula, letting the uncooked eggs flow underneath.
6. Sprinkle crumbled feta cheese over one half of the omelette.
7. Once the eggs are mostly set but still slightly runny on top, carefully fold the omelette in half over the cheese using the spatula.
8. Cook for another 1-2 minutes until the cheese melts, and the omelette is cooked through.
9. Slide the spinach and feta omelette onto a plate.
10. Garnish with sliced avocado on the side.
11. Serve your delicious Spinach and Feta Omelette with Avocado Slices for a nutritious breakfast!

Lunch: Vegan Buddha Bowl with Quinoa and Tahini Dressing

For the Vegan Buddha Bowl:

Ingredients:

- 1 cup cooked quinoa
- 1 cup chickpeas, cooked or canned, drained and rinsed
- 1 cup broccoli florets, steamed
- 1 medium carrot, julienned or grated
- 1/2 cucumber, sliced
- 1/2 avocado, sliced
- 1 cup red cabbage, shredded

- Sesame seeds for garnish
- Fresh cilantro or parsley for garnish

For the Tahini Dressing:

Ingredients:

- 1/4 cup tahini
- 2 tablespoons lemon juice
- 1 tablespoon soy sauce or tamari
- 1 tablespoon maple syrup
- 1 clove garlic, minced
- Water (to thin as needed)
- Salt and pepper to taste

Instructions:

For the Vegan Buddha Bowl:

1. Arrange cooked quinoa, chickpeas, broccoli, carrot, cucumber, avocado, and red cabbage in a bowl.
2. Garnish with sesame seeds and fresh cilantro or parsley.

For the Tahini Dressing:

1. In a bowl, whisk together tahini, lemon juice, soy sauce or tamari, maple syrup, and minced garlic.
2. Add water gradually until the dressing reaches your desired consistency.
3. Season with salt and pepper to taste.

Assembling the Buddha Bowl:

1. Drizzle the tahini dressing over the Vegan Buddha Bowl.
2. Toss gently to coat the ingredients with the dressing.
3. Serve immediately and enjoy your nutritious and flavorful Vegan Buddha Bowl with Quinoa and Tahini Dressing for lunch!

Dinner: Grilled Chicken Caesar Salad with Gluten-Free Croutons

For Grilled Chicken Caesar Salad:

Ingredients:

For the Grilled Chicken:

- 2 boneless, skinless chicken breasts
- 2 tablespoons olive oil
- 1 teaspoon garlic powder
- Salt and black pepper to taste
- Lemon wedges for serving

For the Caesar Salad:

- Romaine lettuce, washed and chopped
- 1/2 cup cherry tomatoes, halved
- 1/4 cup grated vegan Parmesan cheese
- Caesar dressing (store-bought or homemade, see below)
- Gluten-free croutons (store-bought or homemade, see below)

For the Caesar Dressing:

- 1/2 cup vegan mayonnaise
- 2 tablespoons Dijon mustard
- 1 tablespoon capers, minced
- 2 cloves garlic, minced
- 1 tablespoon lemon juice
- 1 teaspoon vegan Worcestershire sauce
- Salt and black pepper to taste

For Gluten-Free Croutons:

- 2 cups gluten-free bread cubes
- 2 tablespoons olive oil
- 1 teaspoon garlic powder
- 1 teaspoon dried thyme
- Salt and black pepper to taste

Instructions:

For the Grilled Chicken:

1. Preheat the grill to medium-high heat.
2. In a bowl, mix olive oil, garlic powder, salt, and black pepper.
3. Rub the chicken breasts with the olive oil mixture.
4. Grill the chicken for 6-8 minutes per side or until cooked through.
5. Let the chicken rest for a few minutes, then slice it into thin strips.

For the Caesar Dressing:

1. In a bowl, whisk together vegan mayonnaise, Dijon mustard, minced capers, minced garlic, lemon juice, vegan Worcestershire sauce, salt, and black pepper.

For Gluten-Free Croutons:

1. Preheat the oven to 375°F (190°C).
2. Toss gluten-free bread cubes with olive oil, garlic powder, dried thyme, salt, and black pepper.
3. Spread the seasoned bread cubes on a baking sheet.
4. Bake in the preheated oven for 10-15 minutes or until the croutons are golden and crispy.

Assembling the Grilled Chicken Caesar Salad:

1. In a large bowl, combine chopped Romaine lettuce, cherry tomatoes, and grated vegan Parmesan cheese.
2. Add the sliced grilled chicken on top.
3. Drizzle Caesar dressing over the salad and toss to coat.
4. Garnish with gluten-free croutons.
5. Serve immediately, and enjoy your hearty and delicious

Friday:

Breakfast: Chia Seed Pudding Parfait with Mango and Coconut Flakes

Ingredients:

For the Chia Seed Pudding:

- 1/4 cup chia seeds
- 1 cup coconut milk (or any plant-based milk)
- 1 tablespoon maple syrup or agave nectar
- 1/2 teaspoon vanilla extract

For the Parfait:

- Chia Seed Pudding
- 1 ripe mango, diced
- Coconut flakes for topping

Instructions:

For the Chia Seed Pudding:

1. In a bowl, whisk together chia seeds, coconut milk, maple syrup (or agave nectar), and vanilla extract.
2. Whisk thoroughly to ensure there are no lumps and the chia seeds are evenly distributed.
3. Let the mixture sit for a few minutes, then whisk again to avoid clumping.
4. Cover the bowl and refrigerate the chia seed pudding for at least 2 hours or overnight to allow it to thicken.

For the Parfait:

1. Once the Chia Seed Pudding has set, layer it in serving glasses or jars.
2. Add a layer of diced ripe mango on top of the chia seed pudding.
3. Repeat the layers until you fill the glasses or jars.
4. Top the parfait with coconut flakes for added texture.
5. Optionally, garnish with additional mango slices or a sprinkle of coconut flakes.

6. Serve and enjoy your refreshing and nutritious Chia Seed Pudding Parfait with Mango and Coconut Flakes for breakfast!

Lunch: Vegetable Stir-Fry with Tofu over Brown Rice

For Vegetable Stir-Fry with Tofu:

Ingredients:

For the Stir-Fry:

- 1 block extra-firm tofu, pressed and cubed
- 2 tablespoons soy sauce or tamari
- 1 tablespoon sesame oil
- 1 tablespoon vegetable oil
- 2 cloves garlic, minced
- 1 tablespoon fresh ginger, grated
- 1 broccoli crown, florets separated
- 1 bell pepper, thinly sliced
- 1 carrot, julienned
- 1 cup snap peas, ends trimmed
- 1 cup sliced mushrooms
- 1 cup baby corn, halved
- 2 green onions, sliced (for garnish)

For the Sauce:

- 3 tablespoons soy sauce or tamari
- 2 tablespoons hoisin sauce
- 1 tablespoon rice vinegar
- 1 tablespoon maple syrup or agave nectar
- 1 teaspoon cornstarch (optional, for thickening)

For Serving:

- Cooked brown rice

Instructions:

For the Tofu:

1. In a bowl, toss the cubed tofu with soy sauce or tamari. Let it marinate for at least 15 minutes.
2. Heat sesame oil and vegetable oil in a large skillet or wok over medium-high heat.
3. Add the marinated tofu to the skillet and cook until golden brown on all sides. Remove tofu from the skillet and set aside.

For the Stir-Fry:

1. In the same skillet, add a bit more oil if needed. Sauté minced garlic and grated ginger until fragrant.
2. Add broccoli, bell pepper, julienned carrot, snap peas, mushrooms, and baby corn. Stir-fry for 5-7 minutes or until vegetables are crisp-tender.
3. Return the cooked tofu to the skillet with the vegetables.

For the Sauce:

1. In a small bowl, whisk together soy sauce or tamari, hoisin sauce, rice vinegar, maple syrup or agave nectar, and cornstarch (if using).
2. Pour the sauce over the tofu and vegetables. Stir well to coat everything evenly. Cook for an additional 2-3 minutes until the sauce thickens.

For Serving:

1. Serve the Vegetable Stir-Fry with Tofu over cooked brown rice.
2. Garnish with sliced green onions.
3. Enjoy your delicious and wholesome Vegetable Stir-Fry with Tofu for lunch!

Dinner: Gluten-Free Margherita Pizza with Mixed Greens Salad

Ingredients:

For the Gluten-Free Pizza Crust:

- 2 cups gluten-free all-purpose flour
- 1 teaspoon baking powder
- 1 teaspoon xanthan gum
- 1/2 teaspoon salt

- 1 cup warm water

- 2 tablespoons olive oil

- 1 teaspoon apple cider vinegar

For the Pizza Toppings:

- 1/2 cup pizza sauce

- 1 1/2 cups fresh mozzarella cheese, sliced

- 2-3 tomatoes, thinly sliced

- Fresh basil leaves

- Olive oil for drizzling

- Salt and black pepper to taste

For the Mixed Greens Salad:

- Mixed salad greens (lettuce, arugula, spinach)

- Cherry tomatoes, halved

- Cucumber, sliced

- Balsamic vinaigrette dressing

Instructions:

For the Gluten-Free Pizza Crust:

1. Preheat the oven to 425°F (220°C).

2. In a bowl, whisk together gluten-free flour, baking powder, xanthan gum, and salt.

3. In a separate bowl, combine warm water, olive oil, and apple cider vinegar.

4. Gradually add the wet ingredients to the dry ingredients, mixing well until a dough forms.

5. Place the dough on a parchment-lined pizza stone or baking sheet.

6. Use your hands to press the dough into a round pizza crust, about 12 inches in diameter.

7. Bake the crust in the preheated oven for 8-10 minutes or until it starts to firm up but is not fully cooked.

For Assembling the Pizza:

1. Remove the partially baked pizza crust from the oven.

2. Spread pizza sauce evenly over the crust.

3. Arrange fresh mozzarella slices and tomato slices on top.

4. Season with salt and black pepper to taste.

5. Return the pizza to the oven and bake for an additional 10-12 minutes or until the cheese is melted and bubbly, and the crust is golden.

6. Remove the pizza from the oven and top with fresh basil leaves.

7. Drizzle with olive oil.

For the Mixed Greens Salad:

1. In a bowl, toss mixed salad greens, cherry tomatoes, and cucumber.

2. Drizzle with balsamic vinaigrette dressing and toss to coat.

For Serving:

1. Slice the Gluten-Free Margherita Pizza and serve it alongside the Mixed Greens Salad.

2. Enjoy your delicious and gluten-free dinner!

Saturday:

Breakfast: Gluten-Free Pancakes with Fresh Berries and Maple Syrup

For Gluten-Free Pancakes:

Ingredients:

- 1 cup gluten-free all-purpose flour
- 1 tablespoon sugar
- 1 teaspoon baking powder
- 1/2 teaspoon baking soda
- 1/4 teaspoon salt
- 1 cup buttermilk (or dairy-free alternative)
- 1 large egg (or egg substitute for vegan option)
- 2 tablespoons melted butter (or melted coconut oil for dairy-free option)
- Fresh berries for topping

- Maple syrup for drizzling

Instructions:

1. In a mixing bowl, whisk together gluten-free flour, sugar, baking powder, baking soda, and salt.
2. In a separate bowl, whisk together buttermilk, egg, and melted butter.
3. Pour the wet ingredients into the dry ingredients and stir until just combined. Be careful not to overmix; some lumps are okay.
4. Let the batter rest for about 5 minutes to allow the gluten-free flour to absorb the liquids.
5. Preheat a griddle or non-stick skillet over medium heat. Lightly grease the surface with oil or butter.
6. Pour 1/4 cup portions of batter onto the griddle for each pancake.
7. Cook until bubbles form on the surface of the pancake and the edges start to set.
8. Flip the pancakes and cook the other side until golden brown.
9. Remove the pancakes from the griddle and repeat with the remaining batter.

For Serving:

1. Stack the gluten-free pancakes on a plate.
2. Top with fresh berries of your choice.
3. Drizzle with maple syrup.
4. Serve warm and enjoy your delightful Gluten-Free Pancakes with Fresh Berries and Maple Syrup for breakfast!

Lunch: Vegan Chickpea Salad Wraps with Lettuce Leaves

For Vegan Chickpea Salad Wraps:

Ingredients:

For the Chickpea Salad:

- 2 cans (15 oz each) chickpeas, drained and rinsed
- 1/2 cup vegan mayonnaise
- 1 tablespoon Dijon mustard

- 1 tablespoon lemon juice
- 2 celery stalks, finely chopped
- 1/4 cup red onion, finely chopped
- 1/4 cup fresh parsley, chopped
- Salt and black pepper to taste

For Wraps:

- Large lettuce leaves (such as Romaine or Bibb)

Optional Toppings:

- Sliced tomatoes
- Avocado slices
- Cucumber strips
- Alfalfa or broccoli sprouts

Instructions:

For the Chickpea Salad:

1. In a large bowl, mash the chickpeas with a fork or potato masher until mostly broken down.
2. Add vegan mayonnaise, Dijon mustard, lemon juice, chopped celery, red onion, fresh parsley, salt, and black pepper.
3. Mix everything together until well combined. Adjust seasoning to taste.

For Assembling the Wraps:

1. Lay a large lettuce leaf flat on a clean surface.
2. Spoon a generous portion of the chickpea salad onto the center of the lettuce leaf.
3. Add your choice of toppings, such as sliced tomatoes, avocado slices, cucumber strips, or sprouts.
4. Fold the sides of the lettuce leaf over the filling, then roll it up tightly to create a wrap.
5. Repeat with the remaining lettuce leaves and chickpea salad.
6. Slice the wraps in half if desired.
7. Serve your Vegan Chickpea Salad Wraps with Lettuce Leaves.

8. Enjoy this light and flavorful lunch option!

Dinner: Lemon Herb Shrimp Skewers with Quinoa Salad

For Lemon Herb Shrimp Skewers:

Ingredients:

- 1 pound large shrimp, peeled and deveined
- 2 tablespoons olive oil
- 2 cloves garlic, minced
- 1 tablespoon fresh lemon juice
- 1 teaspoon lemon zest
- 1 tablespoon fresh parsley, chopped
- 1 teaspoon dried oregano
- Salt and black pepper to taste
- Wooden skewers, soaked in water for 30 minutes

For Quinoa Salad:

Ingredients:

- 1 cup quinoa, rinsed
- 2 cups water or vegetable broth
- 1 cup cherry tomatoes, halved
- 1 cucumber, diced
- 1/4 cup red onion, finely chopped
- 1/4 cup Kalamata olives, sliced
- 1/4 cup feta cheese, crumbled (optional)
- 2 tablespoons fresh lemon juice
- 3 tablespoons olive oil
- 1 tablespoon fresh parsley, chopped
- Salt and black pepper to taste

Instructions:

For Lemon Herb Shrimp Skewers:

1. In a bowl, combine olive oil, minced garlic, lemon juice, lemon zest, chopped parsley, dried oregano, salt, and black pepper.

2. Add the peeled and deveined shrimp to the marinade, ensuring they are well coated. Marinate for at least 15-30 minutes.

3. Preheat the grill or grill pan over medium-high heat.

4. Thread the marinated shrimp onto the soaked wooden skewers.

5. Grill the shrimp skewers for 2-3 minutes per side or until they are opaque and cooked through.

For Quinoa Salad:

1. In a saucepan, combine quinoa and water or vegetable broth. Bring to a boil, then reduce the heat, cover, and simmer for 15-20 minutes or until the quinoa is cooked and liquid is absorbed.

2. Fluff the quinoa with a fork and let it cool to room temperature.

3. In a large bowl, combine cooked quinoa, cherry tomatoes, cucumber, red onion, Kalamata olives, and feta cheese (if using).

4. In a small bowl, whisk together fresh lemon juice, olive oil, chopped parsley, salt, and black pepper.

5. Pour the dressing over the quinoa mixture and toss to combine.

Assembling the Dinner:

1. Serve the Lemon Herb Shrimp Skewers on a plate alongside the Quinoa Salad.

2. Optionally, garnish with additional fresh parsley or lemon wedges.

3. Enjoy your flavorful and wholesome Lemon Herb Shrimp Skewers with Quinoa Salad for dinner!

Sunday:

Breakfast: Vegan Smoothie with Spinach, Banana, and Almond Milk

Vegan Spinach Banana Smoothie:

Ingredients:

- 1 ripe banana
- 1 cup fresh spinach leaves
- 1 cup almond milk (or any plant-based milk)
- 1 tablespoon almond butter (optional)
- Ice cubes (optional)
- 1 tablespoon chia seeds (optional, for added nutrition)
- 1 teaspoon maple syrup or agave nectar (optional, for sweetness)

Instructions:

1. Peel the ripe banana and place it in a blender.
2. Add fresh spinach leaves to the blender.
3. Pour in almond milk.
4. Optionally, add almond butter for a creamier texture.
5. If desired, add ice cubes for a colder and thicker smoothie.
6. For added nutrition, include chia seeds.
7. Optionally, sweeten the smoothie with maple syrup or agave nectar.
8. Blend all the ingredients until smooth and creamy.
9. Pour the vegan spinach banana smoothie into a glass.
10. Optionally, garnish with a sprinkle of chia seeds or a slice of banana.
11. Enjoy your nutritious and refreshing Vegan Smoothie with Spinach, Banana, and Almond Milk for breakfast!

Lunch: Vegan Tofu Stir-Fry with Colorful Vegetables and Rice

Vegan Spinach Banana Smoothie:

Ingredients:

- 1 ripe banana
- 1 cup fresh spinach leaves
- 1 cup almond milk (or any plant-based milk)
- 1 tablespoon almond butter (optional)
- Ice cubes (optional)

- 1 tablespoon chia seeds (optional, for added nutrition)
- 1 teaspoon maple syrup or agave nectar (optional, for sweetness)

Instructions:

1. Peel the ripe banana and place it in a blender.
2. Add fresh spinach leaves to the blender.
3. Pour in almond milk.
4. Optionally, add almond butter for a creamier texture.
5. If desired, add ice cubes for a colder and thicker smoothie.
6. For added nutrition, include chia seeds.
7. Optionally, sweeten the smoothie with maple syrup or agave nectar.
8. Blend all the ingredients until smooth and creamy.
9. Pour the vegan spinach banana smoothie into a glass.
10. Optionally, garnish with a sprinkle of chia seeds or a slice of banana.
11. Enjoy your nutritious and refreshing Vegan Smoothie with Spinach, Banana, and Almond Milk for breakfast!

Dinner: Baked Eggplant Parmesan with Gluten-Free Pasta

Ingredients:

For Baked Eggplant Parmesan:

- 1 large eggplant, thinly sliced
- 1 cup gluten-free breadcrumbs
- 1/2 cup grated vegan Parmesan cheese
- 2 teaspoons dried oregano
- 1 teaspoon dried basil
- 1/2 teaspoon garlic powder
- Salt and black pepper to taste
- 2 cups marinara sauce
- 2 cups vegan mozzarella cheese, shredded
- Fresh basil leaves for garnish (optional)

For Gluten-Free Pasta:

- 8 oz gluten-free pasta of your choice
- Water for boiling
- Salt for pasta water

Instructions:

For Baked Eggplant Parmesan:

1. Preheat the oven to 400°F (200°C).
2. In a bowl, combine gluten-free breadcrumbs, grated vegan Parmesan cheese, dried oregano, dried basil, garlic powder, salt, and black pepper. Mix well.
3. Dip each eggplant slice into the breadcrumb mixture, ensuring both sides are coated.
4. Place the coated eggplant slices on a baking sheet lined with parchment paper.
5. Bake in the preheated oven for 15-20 minutes or until the eggplant slices are golden and crispy.
6. In a baking dish, spread a thin layer of marinara sauce.
7. Arrange a layer of baked eggplant slices on top of the sauce.
8. Sprinkle a portion of vegan mozzarella cheese over the eggplant.
9. Repeat the layers until you run out of ingredients, finishing with a layer of vegan mozzarella on top.
10. Bake for an additional 20-25 minutes or until the cheese is melted and bubbly.
11. Optionally, garnish with fresh basil leaves.

For Gluten-Free Pasta:

1. Bring a large pot of salted water to a boil.
2. Cook the gluten-free pasta according to the package instructions until al dente.
3. Drain the pasta.

For Serving:

1. Serve the Baked Eggplant Parmesan over a bed of gluten-free pasta.
2. Garnish with additional marinara sauce and vegan Parmesan if desired.

3. Enjoy your hearty and gluten-free Baked Eggplant Parmesan with Gluten-Free Pasta for dinner!

DINING OUT SAFELY

1. Research Restaurants: Before going out to eat, look into restaurants that cater to gluten-free diets. Gluten-free options and procedures are frequently discussed in online reviews and on restaurant websites.

2. Take the initiative and phone the restaurant ahead of time. Inquire about gluten-free options and discuss any special dietary requirements or concerns with the staff or chef.

3. Select Naturally Gluten-Free Options: Choose naturally gluten-free dishes such as grilled meats, seafood, salads and vegetables. These have a lower risk of cross-contamination.

4. When ordering, state your dietary limitations carefully and inquire about ingredients and preparation techniques. Avoid cross-contamination in common cooking areas by being explicit.

5. Cross-Contamination: Exercise caution when using shared fryers, cooking surfaces and utensils that may have come into touch with gluten. Inquire if the restaurant has a gluten-free preparation space.

6. Gluten-Free Menu Verification: If a restaurant offers a gluten-free menu, ask the personnel about its dependability. Some establishments may feature a distinct menu but it is critical to confirm that the culinary processes are truly gluten-free.

7. Bring Your Own Snacks: Keep gluten-free snacks on hand especially if you're unsure about the available selections. This guarantees that you have a safe backup in case something goes wrong.

8. Apps and Alliances: Use gluten-free apps and internet platforms to find gluten-free-friendly eateries in your neighborhood. Furthermore, several organizations certify gluten-free facilities, providing an additional layer of assurance.

COMMUNICATING WITH RESTAURANTS

1. Make a Reservation: Before going to the restaurant, make a reservation. This gives you the opportunity to discuss your dietary requirements with the staff or chef allowing them enough time to prepare and fulfill your needs.

2. Make It Clear That You Have Celiac Disease or Gluten Sensitivity: Make it clear that you have Celiac Disease or gluten sensitivity, emphasizing the need of avoiding gluten-containing items and cross-contamination.

3. Pose a Question: Inquire about specific menu items, ingredients and cooking techniques. Inquire whether gluten-free choices are available and whether the kitchen can accommodate dietary changes.

4. Highlight Concerns About Cross-Contamination: Emphasize the need of avoiding cross-contamination. Inquire about separate tools, pans and cooking surfaces for gluten-free cooking. This is critical for people who have Celiac Disease.

5. Inquire about Shared Fryers and Cooking facilities: If applicable, ask about shared fryers and cooking facilities. Fried goods, for example can readily get contaminated if they share cooking equipment with gluten-containing foods.

6. Request a Gluten-Free Menu or selections: Determine whether the restaurant has a gluten-free menu or specialized gluten-free selections. However, always double-check with the personnel to confirm the information is current and correct.

7. Express the Severity of Your Condition: Express the severity of your gluten intolerance or Celiac Disease in a kind manner. This helps the restaurant personnel understand the significance of following your dietary requirements.

8. Show Appreciation: Acknowledge and appreciate the restaurant's efforts to meet your gluten-free needs. This encourages sustained attention to nutritional demands and builds a healthy relationship.

9. Use Allergen Menus: Some restaurants offer allergen menus that list which meals are gluten-free. Use these resources to make your selecting process easier.

10. Check Your Order: When your food arrives, double-check that it meets your gluten-free requirements. If you have any questions or concerns, don't be afraid to ask for clarification.

GLUTEN-FREE FLOURS AND BAKING INGREDIENTS

1. Almond Flour: Ground almonds produce a moist, nutty flour that may be used in a number of baked items.
2. Coconut Flour: This flour has a subtle coconut flavor and is strong in fiber. It is frequently combined with other gluten-free flours.
3. Rice Flour (Brown and White): Rice flour is a versatile gluten-free baking ingredient. Brown rice flour imparts a nutty flavor, whilst white rice flour is milder.
4. Quinoa Flour: Quinoa flour provides a protein boost and works well in both sweet and savory recipes.
5. Buckwheat Flour: Contrary to popular belief, buckwheat flour is gluten-free. Buckwheat flour has a particular flavor and works well in pancakes, crepes and bread.
6. Sorghum Flour: Made from sorghum grain, this flour has a moderate flavor and can be used in place of wheat flour in a variety of recipes.
7. Tapioca Flour/Starch: Adds lightness and texture to gluten-free baked items. It is frequently combined with other flours.
8. Arrowroot flour acts as a thickening agent and can help baked foods have a lighter texture.
9. Potato starch: A fine, white powder that adds softness and suppleness to gluten-free baked goods.
10. Cornflour: A thickening agent that can also be found in gluten-free flour blends.
11. Chickpea Flour (Garbanzo Bean Flour): High in protein, this flour is widely used in savory recipes such as socca and chickpea pancakes.

12. Xanthan Gum: A gluten-free baking binder that mimics the flexibility of gluten. Many recipes rely on it to provide the desired texture.
13. Psyllium Husk: Increases the moisture and structure of gluten-free breads and baked items.
14. Gluten-Free Baking Powder: Make sure it's clearly labeled gluten-free to avoid cross-contamination.

CHAPTER 10: TRAVELING WITH CELIAC DISEASE

1. Prior to your vacation, investigate gluten-free food choices at your location. Look for gluten-free-friendly restaurants, grocery stores and markets.

2. Pack Gluten-Free Snacks: For the travel, bring a stash of gluten-free snacks. This ensures that you have safe options when your immediate gluten-free options are restricted.

3. Notify Airlines and Accommodations: When booking your flight, advise the airline of your dietary limitations. Similarly, notify hotels or accommodations in advance so that required arrangements can be made.

4. Translation Cards: Make or receive gluten-free dining cards in your destination's language. These cards can be used to clearly express your dietary preferences to restaurant staff.

5. Download Gluten-Free applications: Use mobile applications to learn about gluten-free dining options. These apps frequently offer ratings and reviews from other travelers.

6. Communication is essential: When dining out, inform the restaurant personnel of your gluten-free requirements. Explain the significance of avoiding gluten due to Celiac Disease.

7. Maintain Knowledge of Local food: Become acquainted with the local food and common ingredients. This information allows you to make more educated decisions and locate naturally gluten-free solutions.

8. seek for Gluten-Free Certifications: When purchasing packaged foods from other countries, seek for gluten-free certifications or labels. This ensures that the product complies with gluten-free requirements.

9. Gluten-Free Pantry Essentials: Pack gluten-free pantry products such as gluten-free pasta, snacks, and sauces in your luggage. This guarantees that you have options that are both familiar and safe.

10. Prepare for Language Barriers: Learn important terms in the local language pertaining to your dietary needs. This can help you properly convey your requirements.

PACKABLE GLUTEN-FREE SNACKS

1. Almonds, walnuts, sunflower seeds and pumpkin seeds are protein-rich and convenient snacks.
2. Gluten-Free Granola Bars: Look for gluten-free granola bars. They come in a variety of flavors and are ideal for a rapid energy boost.
3. Dried Fruits: For a delicious and filling snack, pack individually portioned packets of dried fruits such as apricots, raisins or apple slices.
4. Rice Cakes: Rice cakes are light and adaptable, and can be eaten on its own or spread with nut butter for a more satisfying option.
5. Popcorn: A gluten-free whole grain snack is air-popped popcorn. Season it with your favorite gluten-free seasonings if desired.
6. Gluten-Free Pretzels: There are numerous gluten-free pretzel options. A little bag is ideal for a crunchy and savory snack.
7. Fresh Fruit: Apples, bananas and oranges are long-lasting fruits that can be readily crushed while traveling.
8. Individually wrapped cheese sticks or cubes are a quick and easy source of protein.
9. Gluten-Free Trail Mix: Mix together nuts, seeds and gluten-free dried fruits to make your own trail mix.
10. Gluten-Free Crackers: For a delightful crunch, choose gluten-free crackers manufactured with alternative flours. They go well with cheese or nut butter.
11. Greek Yoghurt Cups: For a protein-rich snack, grab single-serving cups of gluten-free Greek yogurt if refrigeration is available.
12. Hard-Boiled Eggs: Boil eggs ahead of time and store them in a container for a portable, protein-rich snack.

13. Sliced carrots, cucumbers, or bell peppers are paired with individual servings of gluten-free hummus in this recipe.

14. Beef Jerky: For a handy and savory protein snack, choose gluten-free beef or turkey jerky. Almonds, walnuts, sunflower seeds and pumpkin seeds are protein-rich and convenient snacks.

15. Gluten-Free Granola Bars: Look for gluten-free granola bars. They come in a variety of flavors and are ideal for a rapid energy boost.

16. Dried Fruits: For a delicious and filling snack, pack individually portioned packets of dried fruits such as apricots, raisins or apple slices.

17. Rice Cakes: Rice cakes are light and adaptable, and can be eaten on its own or spread with nut butter for a more satisfying option.

18. Popcorn: A gluten-free whole grain snack is air-popped popcorn. Season it with your favourite gluten-free seasonings if desired.

19. Gluten-Free Pretzels: There are numerous gluten-free pretzel options. A little bag is ideal for a crunchy and savory snack.

20. Fresh Fruit: Apples, bananas and oranges are long-lasting fruits that can be readily crushed while traveling.

21. Individually wrapped cheese sticks or cubes are a quick and easy source of protein.

22. Gluten-Free Trail Mix: Mix together nuts, seeds, and gluten-free dried fruits to make your own trail mix.

23. Gluten-Free Crackers: For a delightful crunch, choose gluten-free crackers manufactured with alternative flours. They go well with cheese or nut butter.

24. Greek Yoghurt Cups: For a protein-rich snack, grab single-serving cups of gluten-free Greek yogurt if refrigeration is available.

25. Hard-Boiled Eggs: Boil eggs ahead of time and store them in a container for a portable, protein-rich snack.

26. Sliced carrots, cucumbers, or bell peppers are paired with individual servings of gluten-free hummus in this recipe.

27. Beef Jerky: For a handy and savory protein snack, choose gluten-free beef or turkey jerky.

ENSURING A BALANCED GLUTEN-FREE DIET

1. Diversify Gluten-Free Grains: To ensure a varied range of nutrients, experiment with gluten-free grains such as quinoa, brown rice, millet and buckwheat.

2. Include Fruits and Vegetables: Eat a variety of colorful fruits and vegetables to acquire critical vitamins, minerals and antioxidants. These foods also help with fiber intake.

3. Choose Lean Proteins: Include lean protein sources including poultry, fish, eggs, lentils and tofu in your diet. These foods promote muscle health and keep you feeling full.

4. Include Dairy or Dairy Alternatives: To achieve calcium and vitamin D requirements, include dairy or fortified dairy alternatives if tolerated. Almond or soy milk are frequently available in gluten free variants.

5. Embrace Healthy Fats: Include sources of healthy fats such as avocados, nuts, seeds, and olive oil in your diet. These fats help with heart health and satiety.

6. Carefully read the labels: Ensure that packaged gluten-free products are not just gluten-free but also nutritious. Some gluten-free options may be deficient in some nutrients, so choose carefully.

7. Sugar and Processed meals to Avoid: Be wary of additional sugars and processed meals in gluten-free items. To promote balanced nutrition, choose whole, minimally processed meals.

8. Maintain Adequate Hydration: Adequate hydration is critical for general health. Drink plenty of water and experiment with herbal teas and naturally flavored water for variation.

9. Consider Nutritional Supplements: If necessary, contact with a healthcare expert to establish whether supplements such as vitamins or minerals, are required to address any potential nutrient gaps in your diet.

10. Plan Balanced Meals: Make a point of eating balanced meals that include a range of proteins, carbohydrates, healthy fats and veggies. Planning ahead of time can help you make healthier decisions.

11. Play with Gluten-Free Superfoods: For added nutritional benefits, incorporate nutrient-dense superfoods such as chia seeds, flaxseeds and hemp seeds into your meals.

COMMON NUTRIENT DEFICIENCIES IN CELIAC PATIENTS

1. Iron malabsorption in the small intestine can result in anemia which causes fatigue, weakness and pale complexion.

2. Calcium: Small intestine damage may impair calcium absorption, affecting bone health and raising the risk of osteoporosis.

3. Calcium absorption is tightly linked to vitamin D, and celiac disease patients may be deficient in vitamin D. This deficit can have an impact on bone health as well as overall immunological function.

4. Folate (Vitamin B9): Malabsorption can result in a folate shortage, affecting red blood cell formation and potentially causing anemia.

5. Vitamin B12: Damage to the small intestine can impair vitamin B12 absorption, resulting in anemia and neurological problems.

6. Zinc: Celiac disease can reduce zinc absorption, which can compromise immune function, wound healing and skin health.

7. Magnesium deficiency can result from malabsorption, which can cause muscle cramps, weakness and abnormal heart beats.

8. Phosphorus: Phosphorus absorption may be reduced, affecting bone health and energy metabolism.

9. Potassium deficiency can impact potassium levels, causing muscle weakness, weariness and electrolyte abnormalities.

10. Thiamine (Vitamin B1) deficiency: Thiamine deficiency can disrupt nerve function and cause symptoms such as tingling or numbness.

www.ingramcontent.com/pod-product-compliance
Lightning Source LLC
Chambersburg PA
CBHW070928260726

48661CB00003B/876